W. Clayman

Hyperlipidaemia
IN
PRACTICE

David J Galton MSc MD FRCP

Professor of Human Metabolism
St Bartholomew's Hospital
London, UK

Wilhelm Krone MD

Professor and Chairman
2nd Department of Medicine
University of Cologne
Cologne, Germany

Gower Medical Publishing · **LONDON · NEW YORK**

Distributed in the USA and Canada by:
J B Lippincott Company
East Washington Square
Philadelphia
PA 19105
USA

Distributed in the UK and Continental Europe by:
Gower Medical Publishing
Middlesex House
34–42 Cleveland Street
London W1P 5FB
UK

Distributed in Australia and New Zealand by:
Harper and Row (Australia) Pty Ltd
PO Box 226
Artarmon
NSW 2064
AUSTRALIA

Distributed in Southeast Asia, Hong Kong, India and Pakistan by:
Harper and Row (Asia) Pte Ltd
37 Jalan Pemimpin 02–01
Singapore 2057

Distributed in Japan by:
Nankodo Co Ltd
42–6 Hongo 3-chome
Bunkyo-ku
Tokyo 113
JAPAN

Project Manager:	Saba Zafar
Designer:	Balvir Koura
Illustrators:	Robert Wilkins
	Dereck Johnson
	David McElwaine
	Mark Willey
	Lee Smith
	Marion Tasker
Page layout:	Michel Laake

British Library Cataloguing in Publication Data:
Galton, D.J. (David Jeremy)
Hyperlipidaemia in practice.
1. Humans. Hyperlipidaemia
I. Title II. Krone, Wilhelm
616.3997

Library of Congress Cataloging in Publication Data:
Galton, David J.
Hyperlipidaemia in practice/David J. Galton, Wilhelm Krone.
p. cm.
Includes index.
1. Hyperlipidemia. I. Krone, Wilhelm. II. Title.
[DNLM: 1. Hyperlipidemia. WD 200.5.H8 G181h]
RC632.H87G35 1991
616.3'997--dc20
DLC
for Library of Congress

ISBN: 0–397–44762–0

Text set in Bembo and Futura

Typesetting by M to N Typesetting, London

Produced by Chroma Graphics, Singapore

Printed and bound in Hong Kong

©Copyright 1991 (Text and photographs) by David J Galton, and (Diagrammatic illustrations) by Gower Medical Publishing, 34–42 Cleveland Street, London W1P 5FB, England. All rights reserved. No part of this publication may be reproduced, stored in a retrieval system or transmitted in any form or by any means electronic, mechanical, photocopying, recording or otherwise, without prior written permission of the publisher.
The right of David J Galton and Wilhelm Krone to be identified as authors of this work has been asserted by them in accordance with the Copyright, Designs and Patents Act 1988.

Preface

This book describes some of the practical problems that arise when managing patients with lipid disorders, and sets out the theoretical background to the subject. It provides an introduction for those wanting to learn about this complex and often confusing area of clinical medicine. The use of an atlas approach was designed to get away from the intricate terminology that has grown up around the subject and to avoid a text interspersed with long lists of abbreviations. Whenever possible, pictures of clinical cases are presented, and diagrams have been made as simple as possible, not we hope, at the expense of accuracy, but by omitting unnecessary detail.

This book is intended for doctors who want to set up, or have just started a lipid clinic, either in general practice (such as the Diabetic Miniclinics) or in hospital practice in association with departments of Chemical Pathology or General Medicine.

The location of the Lipid Clinic at St Bartholomew's Hospital, a general hospital in Central London with busy Diabetic, Cardiac, and Cardiothoracic Departments, has clearly influenced the range of patients and types of problems that are described. Furthermore, strong links with Moorfields Eye Hospital may account for the greater variety of eye complications than other lipid clinics would perhaps encounter.

This book would not have been written but for the support and referral from consultant colleagues in Cardiology (Drs R Spurrell, S Banim, D Tunstall–Pedoe, D Dymond, and A Nathan); in Cardiothoracic Surgery (Mr G Rees and Mr S Edmondson); and in Endocrinology and Diabetes (Professors GM Besser and J AH Wass, and Dr E Gale), to mention and thank just a few.

Many of the patients described in this book have been studied extensively, and their case histories have been published in collaboration with previous colleagues at St Bartholomew's Hospital; we are particularly indebted to Drs JPD Reckless, G Jerums, G Holdsworth, DJ Betteridge, KG Taylor, P Clifton–Bligh, PM Dodson, A Rees, N Jowett, G Hitman, M Vella, D Thomas, and J Stocks for their enthusiastic efforts in the field. We are also extremely grateful to Drs J V Anderson, MG Baroni, JC Alcolado, and C Galton for their unflagging search for errors in text and figures. Sue Goddard provided prompt and cheerful secretarial services in the face of the numerous alterations and revisions.

Our editor, Saba Zafar, and designer, Balvir Koura, without whom this work would not be possible, are responsible for the fine quality of the illustrations and layout.

DAVID J GALTON, London
WILHELM KRONE, Cologne
1991

Foreword

Drs Galton and Krone are to be commended for putting together *Hyperlipidaemia in Practice*, a concise, yet thorough compendium of up-to-date knowledge about the pathophysiology, genetics, diagnosis, and treatment of common lipid disorders seen in clinical practice. The case histories serve to focus attention on some of the major issues. The remarkable number of simple and clear illustrations adds to the lucidity of the text, while accuracy is not sacrificed.

I have known Dr Galton for more than 20 years and have valued our collegial interchanges about issues relating to human hyperlipidaemic disorders. I plan on using some of these illustrations for my own teaching slides, which should be just as valuable in North America as they are likely to be in Europe.

This book should be a very worthwhile addition to the active library of any practitioner involved in the care of patients with lipid disorders.

EDWIN L BIERMAN
Seattle, Washington, USA

To our long-suffering patients

Acknowledgements

We would like to thank the following for providing illustrative material: Dr G Enzi, Padua, Italy (Fig. 2.51); Dr PN Durrington, Manchester, UK (Fig. 2.10); Dr JPD Reckless, Bath, UK (Fig. 1.7); Dr RO Scow, Bethesda, USA (Fig. 1.32); and Dr GM Reaven, Palo Alto, USA (Fig. 8.7).

Other photographs have been taken by the Department of Medical Illustration under the excellent directorship of Peter Cull at St Bartholomew's Hospital, London; we are most indebted to all in the Department for their dedicated skill and service.

Contents

THE CHEMISTRY OF LIPIDS	1
INHERITED DEFECTS OF LIPID METABOLISM	24
THE NEW LIPIDS	46
EPIDEMIOLOGY OF BLOOD LIPIDS AND ATHEROSCLEROSIS	66
COMPLICATIONS OF HYPERLIPIDAEMIA IN THE EYE	70
COMPLICATIONS OF HYPERLIPIDAEMIA AT THE ARTERIAL WALL	84
SECONDARY HYPERLIPIDAEMIAS	93
THERAPY	104
INTERVENTION TRIALS	120
THE LIPID CLINIC	127
FURTHER READING	132
INDEX	134

CHAPTER ONE

The Chemistry of Lipids

THE MOLECULES

The fats or lipids are not a single class of chemical compounds, as are the proteins or nucleic acids. Triglycerides (Fig. 1.1) and phospholipids (Fig. 1.2) form a family of molecules which have varying lengths of long-chain fatty acids attached to the head of the molecule (for example, glycerol for triglycerides, and phosphatidylcholine for a phospholipid). Cholesterol is a steroid molecule

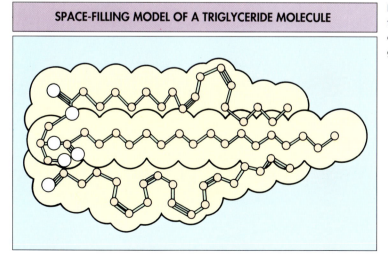

Fig. 1.1 The structure of a triglyceride molecule. Three long-chain fatty acids are attached to glycerol.

SPACE-FILLING MODEL OF A TRIGLYCERIDE MOLECULE

The Chemistry of Lipids

related more to cortisone, aldosterone, and the bile salts than to triglycerides or phospholipids (Fig. 1.3). However, the fats share two common properties: insolubility in water, and solubility in solvents such as chloroform or ether. Fats are water insoluble because they possess long chains of hydrocarbons that have very little electrical charge, thus dispersion in water is not easily achieved; this makes it very difficult to transport fats in the bloodstream. An efficient, but complex lipid-transport system has evolved to circumvent this problem.

Despite the problems of water insolubility and transport, the fats make an excellent fuel system, and are good particularly for storing energy since their calorie value (kcal/g) is more than twice that of carbohydrates. The long-chain fatty acids of triglycerides (and to a lesser extent, phospholipids)

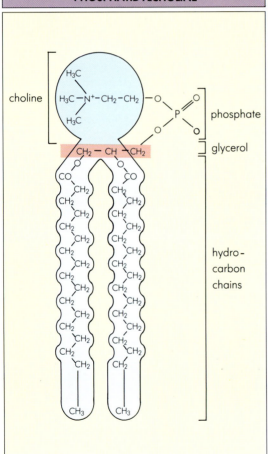

Fig. 1.2 The structure of a phospholipid molecule. This is the primary structural element in all cell membranes. Four main types of phospholipids are found in cell membranes. The phospholipid shown is phosphatidylcholine. The other three phospholipids differ from phosphatidylcholine, and from one another, only in the chemical structure of their head groups.

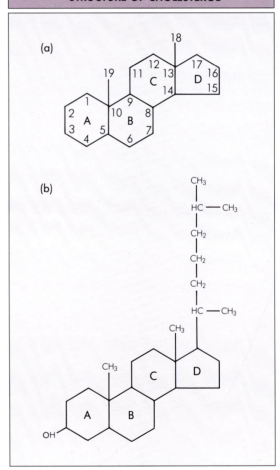

Fig. 1.3 The ring structure of cholesterol. This structure is quite unlike that of the two other lipid classes. (a) The general ring structure for a steroid molecule. (b) Addition of a hydrocarbon chain at carbon 17 completes the structure for cholesterol.

are primarily fuel molecules. In contrast, cholesterol and phospholipids are major structural components of cell membranes, allowing compartmentation of the aqueous environment of the cell into mitochondrial, cytoplasmic, and nuclear spaces.

LIPIDS AS FUELS: STORAGE

The main storage fuels of the body are triglycerides (Fig. 1.4). Triglycerides pack down in a semi-crystalline array, excluding water, and occupy less space per gram weight than glycogen. Glycogen

CHAIN PACKING OF TRIGLYCERIDE MOLECULES

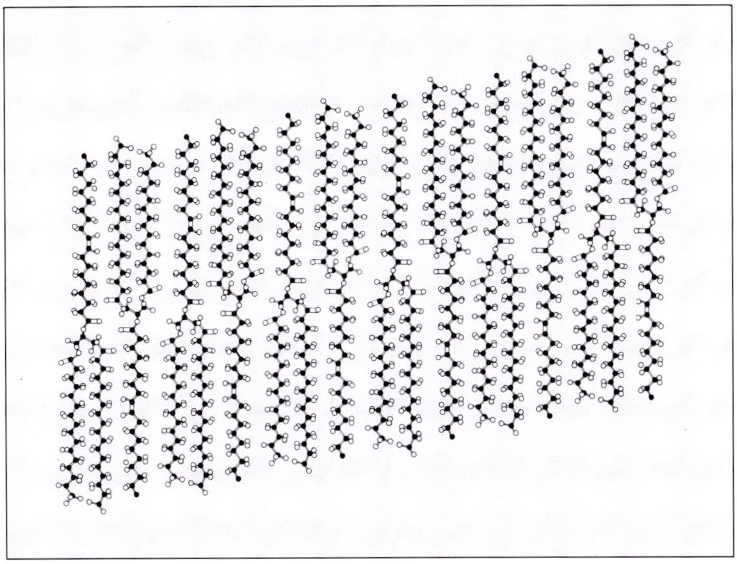

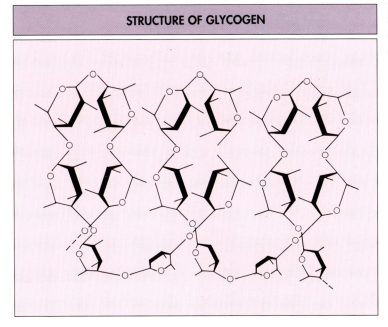

Fig. 1.4 A two-dimensional representation of chain packing of triglyceride molecules. In reality, there is a solid three-dimensional packing which gives rise to a crystalline-like array.

STRUCTURE OF GLYCOGEN

Fig. 1.5 A possible structure of the amylase chain of glycogen. Glycogen is seen here as a polymer of glucose residues.

The Chemistry of Lipids

forms a globular network of glucose molecules which traps water, and constitutes a less-efficient fuel store than the triglycerides (Fig. 1.5). On average, an individual may store 10kg of triglyceride in adipose tissue compared to 150g of glycogen in the liver (Fig. 1.6).

The adipose cell plays a key role in lipid metabolism. Its histology may suggest an inert storage cell, but this would belie its appearance (Fig. 1.7). It is in fact metabolically very active and is a main site of glucose and fatty-acid interconversions which involve triglyceride synthesis and breakdown (Fig. 1.8).

The breakdown of adipocyte triglycerides is under hormonal control and regulates the release of free fatty acids into the blood, depending on the caloric requirements of other tissues such as muscle or heart. Glycerol is also released and circulates back to the liver for re-synthesis of glucose via the pathways of gluconeogenesis; the adipose cell thus has glycerol as an alternative 'glucose' store. The release of fatty acids and glycerol occurs mainly in the fasting state in order to supply other tissues such as heart, skeletal muscle, and the kidneys, with substrates for oxidation. This release is suppressed in the fed state when there is a plentiful supply of nutrients available from the intestines.

		STORAGE FUELS IN A NORMAL MALE (70kg)	
		Triglycerides	**Glycogen**
	Storage site	Adipose cell	Liver, muscle cell
	Quantity stored	10kg	0.15kg
Fuel types	Fatty acids	9kg	
	Glucose as glycerol	0.5kg	0.15kg
	Calorie value	9.5kcal/g	4.2kcal/g

Fig. 1.6 Storage fuels in a normal 70-kg male.

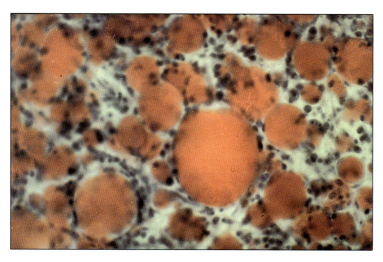

Fig. 1.7 Low-power view of adipocytes stained with oil-red O. Although the cells appear to be filled with fat vacuoles, they are metabolically very active.

Lipids as Fuels: Transport

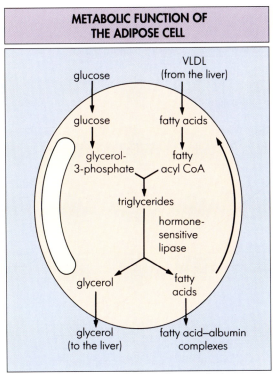

Fig. 1.8 The major metabolic pathways of adipose cells involve uptake of glucose and fatty acids derived from VLDL, their interconversions to triglycerides, and release of fatty acids and glycerol from stores of triglycerides (which is under hormonal control).

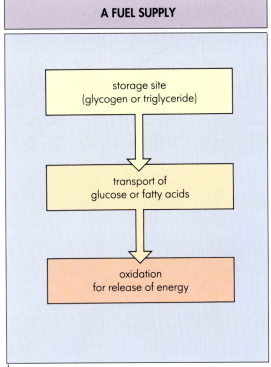

Fig. 1.9 A simplified scheme for a fuel supply. In man, the major storage sites are adipose tissue and liver, and the major oxidation sites are muscle, heart, and other peripheral tissues.

LIPIDS AS FUELS: TRANSPORT

The basic elements of a simple fuel supply include storage, transport, and oxidation for release of energy (Fig. 1.9). The fats are excellent storage fuels, but are difficult to transport due to their insolubility in water. Fatty acids circulate as a complex with albumin, and constitute an important immediate supply of energy, although they were not recognized as circulating fuels for a long time. Although their concentration in plasma is ten-fold lower than glucose, their turnover time is seven times greater than glucose (Fig. 1.10), providing a calorie supply equivalent to that of

A COMPARISON OF SEVERAL PLASMA FUELS				
Fuel	Plasma concentration		Plasma half-life	Calorie supply
Glucose	100 mg/dl	5.5 mM	20 min	0.3 kcal/min
Free fatty acids	10–15 mg/dl	0.4–0.6 mM	3 min	4.4 kcal/min
Triglycerides	150 mg/dl	1.8 mM	180 min	

Fig. 1.10 A comparison of the concentrations and energy supplies of several plasma fuels.

The Chemistry of Lipids

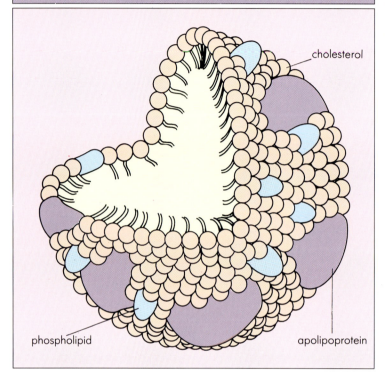

Fig. 1.11 A simplified scheme of the surface components of a lipoprotein particle. The outer shell contains cholesterol, phospholipids, and apolipoproteins, to allow stabilization of the particle structure in plasma.

glucose. If the concentration of fatty acids is too high, metabolic acidosis will result. For this reason, fatty acids circulate in an esterified form as triglycerides, which require the development of the lipoprotein system for their transport in the bloodstream.

Lipoproteins

Lipoproteins are designed to transport triglyceride and cholesterol from the intestines and liver for use in peripheral tissues as oxidizable fuel, and to form apolar (less electrically charged) molecules which are required for the assembly and maintenance of cell membranes. Lipoproteins are complex aggregates of lipid and protein molecules, which are sufficiently stable to form particles for circulation in plasma. A complicated group of proteins, enzymes, and receptors have evolved to optimize the transport and delivery of fat in these particles to peripheral tissues. Unfortunately, this often breaks down and gives rise to the common disorders of lipid transport (hyperlipidaemias) and lipid storage (particularly atherosclerosis).

The structure of lipoproteins

The lipoprotein particle consists of an outer shell of phospholipids and cholesterol in which various peptide components (the apolipoproteins) are embedded. This outer shell stabilizes the particle in the aqueous environment of plasma (Fig. 1.11). Some of the peptides carry sites for receptor recognition to allow uptake of the particle into cells; others can activate enzymes involved in the breakdown of the particle for release of its lipid load. The core of the particle carries the lipid load as triglycerides in the case of chylomicrons, very low-density lipoproteins (VLDL), or intermediate-density lipoproteins (IDL); as cholesterol, in the case of low-density lipoproteins (LDL); and as phospholipids, in the case of high-density lipoproteins (HDL) (Figs. 1.12 and 1.13). The particle size will clearly vary depending on the nature and quantity of the lipid core. The triglyceride-rich

Lipids as Fuels: Transport

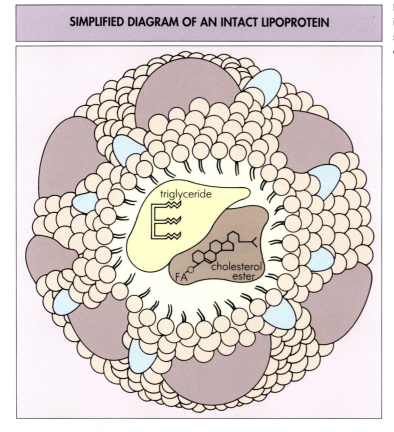

Fig. 1.12 A simplified diagram of an intact lipoprotein particle showing surface and core components of cholesterol and triglyceride.

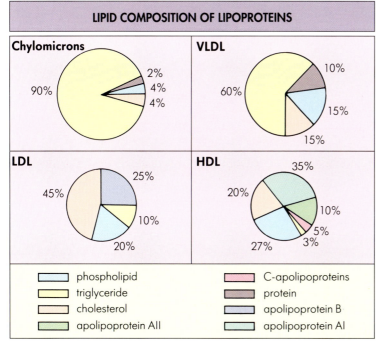

Fig. 1.13 Pye diagrams showing the lipid composition of the various lipoprotein classes.

The Chemistry of Lipids

particles (chylomicrons and VLDL) are larger than the cholesterol-rich particles (LDL) (Fig. 1.14). The size of the particle and its lipid composition affects its buoyant density or flotation rates in salt solutions. This allows separation of the main classes of lipoproteins into chylomicrons, VLDL, LDL, and HDL, by means of density-gradient centrifugation.

Lipoprotein (a)

An extraordinary lipoprotein, lipoprotein (a), has recently been discovered (Fig. 1.15). This consists of the cholesterol-rich lipoprotein, LDL, attached to a long repeated chain of a structure known as kringle 4. Such a kringle is also found in plasminogen, and the term kringle arises because of its supposed resemblance to a pretzel. Plasminogen is part of the fibrinolytic system and is converted to the enzyme, plasmin. Plasmin breaks down fibrin and assists in the dissolution of a thrombus. Why a component of plasminogen should be found attached to a cholesterol-rich lipoprotein, defies explanation at present. However, elevated levels of lipoprotein (a) have been found in patients with premature coronary artery disease, suggesting that it may in some way interfere with the normal

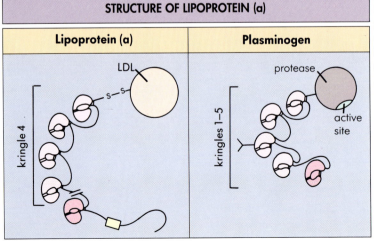

Fig. 1.14 The relationship of the size of various lipoprotein particles with flotation rates in an ultracentrifuge.

Fig. 1.15 The structure of lipoprotein (a) showing its relationship with plasminogen. The fourth kringle of plasminogen is repeated in lipoprotein (a) and attached by disulphide linkage to apolipoprotein B of LDL.

function of plasminogen at the endothelial lining of arteries to remove small fibrin deposits and may subsequently promote thrombosis.

Identification of lipoproteins

DENSITY-GRADIENT CENTRIFUGATION

Lipoproteins can be separated into various classes by two basic techniques — centrifugation or electrophoresis. In the technique of density-gradient centrifugation (Fig. 1.16), a density gradient, for example of sodium chloride, is established in a centrifuge tube (Fig. 1.16a) and the lipoproteins (in serum) are subsequently layered at the bottom of the tube (Fig. 1.16b). After the tube is spun in a centrifuge (Fig. 1.16c), the particles of the lightest buoyant density (chylomicrons) float to the top; the triglyceride-rich lipoproteins (VLDL) also float to their equivalent density band (halfway up the tube) (Fig. 1.16d). The cholesterol-rich particles (LDL), which are heavier, form a band lower down in the tube (Fig. 1.16d), whilst HDL sink to the bottom of the tube. The various bands which are collected after puncturing the bottom of the tube, give rise to the lipoprotein profile (Fig. 1.17).

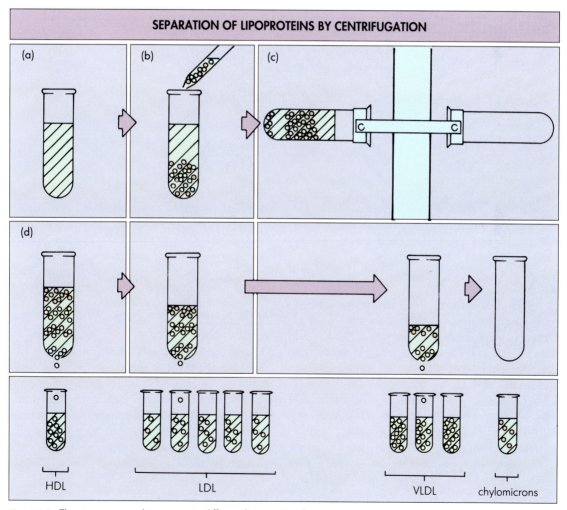

Fig. 1.16 The steps required to separate different lipoprotein classes according to buoyant densities by density-gradient centrifugation (see text for explanation of the steps involved).

The Chemistry of Lipids

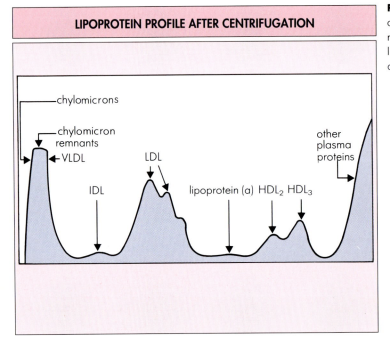

Fig. 1.17 Distribution of the main classes of plasma lipoproteins of a normolipidaemic human subject. The lipoproteins were separated by density-gradient centrifugation.

If the density gradient is adjusted so that the chylomicrons and VLDL float together, a single peak will result and HDL will come out as two fractions, HDL_2 and HDL_3 (Fig. 1.17).

ELECTROPHORESIS
In electrophoresis, the lipoproteins are layered onto a support medium such as cellulose acetate, and are then subjected to an electric field for several hours (Fig. 1.18). The particles move in the electric field depending on their surface charge and size, and on the pore size of the supporting medium. Chylomicrons remain at the site of application, LDL (β-lipoproteins) migrate into the medium, VLDL (pre-β-lipoproteins) migrate further into the medium, and the smallest particles, HDL (α-lipoproteins), move further towards the anode. The technique of lipoprotein separation by electrophoresis corresponds well to that of density-gradient centrifugation (Fig. 1.19). This accounts for the dual nomenclature of lipoproteins: VLDL, also known as pre-β-lipoproteins; LDL, also known as β-lipoproteins; and HDL, also known as α-lipoproteins. However, the terminology which is now preferred is VLDL, LDL, and HDL, since density-gradient centrifugation provides a better, and more sensitive separation of the lipoprotein classes than electrophoretic techniques.

The composition of lipoproteins

LIPID COMPOSITION
The triglyceride content of lipoproteins decreases steadily from 90% in chylomicrons, to 3% in HDL (see *Fig. 1.13*). Conversely, the phospholipid content increases from 4% in chylomicrons, to 27% in HDL. The decreasing content of triglycerides from chylomicrons to HDL largely accounts for the differences in buoyant densities of these lipoproteins.

PEPTIDE COMPOSITION
The peptide composition of the lipoproteins also varies considerably amongst the classes, although in no regular way. The main component peptides

Lipids as Fuels: Transport

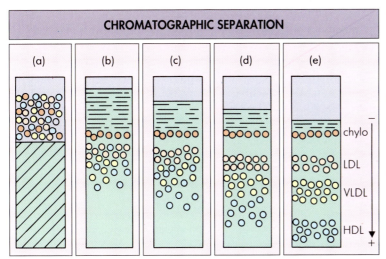

Fig. 1.18 Chromatographic separation of lipoproteins on cellulose acetate. (a) A solution containing a mixture of the lipoproteins is layered onto the cellulose acetate. (b)–(e) The electric field causes separation of the particles by electric charge and particle size, into four bands. Chylomicrons remain at the origin, LDL move into the gel slightly, VLDL move in further, and HDL migrate the furthest.

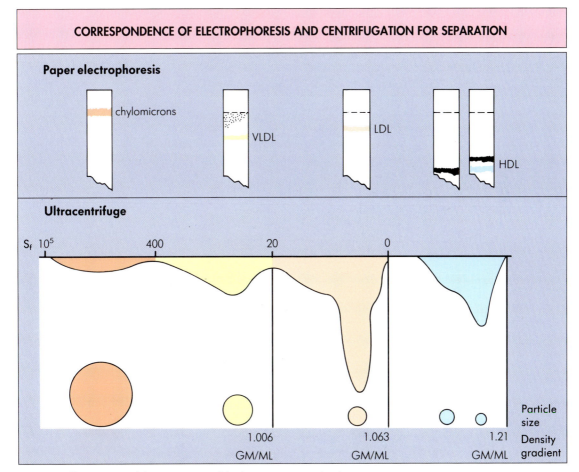

Fig. 1.19 Comparison of the separation of the lipoprotein particles by electrophoresis and density-gradient centrifugation. The correspondence of lipoprotein separation by both methods is good.

of each lipoprotein are illustrated in Fig. 1.20; it should be noted that LDL probably contains only one molecule/particle of apolipoprotein B, but several molecules of apolipoprotein E. Properties of the individual peptides and their possible functions are presented in Fig. 1.21. One notable feature of the B-100 peptide is that it contains a domain for binding to the LDL receptor of peripheral cells, and mutations at this site can interfere with the removal of LDL-cholesterol from plasma. The apolipoprotein-CII peptide is an essential activator of the enzyme, lipoprotein lipase, and defects of this peptide can interfere with the removal of triglyceride-rich lipoproteins from plasma. The normal appearance of some of the C-apolipoproteins after separation by gel electrophoresis, is presented in Fig. 1.22.

Fig. 1.20 The peptide composition of lipoproteins. The major classes of apolipoproteins (A, B, and C) are distributed assymetrically amongst the different lipoproteins.

PROPERTIES OF HUMAN APOLIPOPROTEINS

Apolipo-proteins	Molecular weight	Number of residues	Site of synthesis	Function
AI	28,300	243	intestine liver	activates LCAT
AII	17,000	154	liver intestine	structural
B100	550,000	4,536	liver	binds to LDL receptor
B48	264,000	2,152	intestine	
CI	6,600	57	liver	activates LCAT
CII	8,850	78	liver	activates LPL
CIII	8,800	79	liver	?inhibits LPL
E2, E3, E4	34,000	299	liver intestine	binds to E receptors

LCAT = lecithin:cholesterol acyltransferase; LPL = lipoprotein lipase.

Fig. 1.21 Properties of human apolipoproteins.

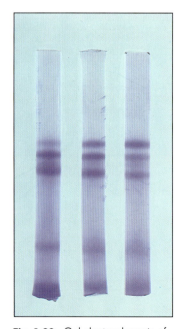

Fig. 1.22 Gel electrophoresis of some C-apolipoproteins showing three bands which consist of apolipoprotein CII, apolipoprotein CIII-1, and apolipoprotein CIII-2 (top to bottom).

Lipids as Fuels: Transport

Origins of lipoproteins

SOURCES OF VERY LOW-DENSITY LIPOPROTEINS

The triglyceride-rich lipoproteins originate from the intestine and liver. Dietary fat is broken down to fatty acids and partial glycerides in the small intestine by the action of pancreatic and intestinal lipases. During absorption through the mucosal wall of the gut, fatty acids and partial glycerides are re-synthesized to triglyceride for packaging into chylomicrons for transport through the lymphatic ducts into the bloodstream (Fig. 1.23). Endogenous fat, which is synthesized in the liver from glucose and fatty acids, is secreted into the bloodstream as VLDL. Small chylomicrons are virtually indistinguishable from large-sized VLDL, the quantity of triglyceride per particle varying with the nutritional and hormonal status at the time of synthesis. During their circulation, triglyceride-rich lipoproteins are gradually delipidated by the action of lipolytic enzymes (lipoprotein lipase and hepatic lipase) and converted through IDL into cholesterol-rich lipoproteins (LDL). This lipolytic cascade involves the conversion of VLDL to LDL (Fig. 1.24). During this conversion, some particles can be removed directly by binding to cell receptors such as the LDL receptor or remnant receptors.

Fig. 1.23 Source of triglyceride-rich lipoproteins and their appearance, as separated by paper electrophoresis.

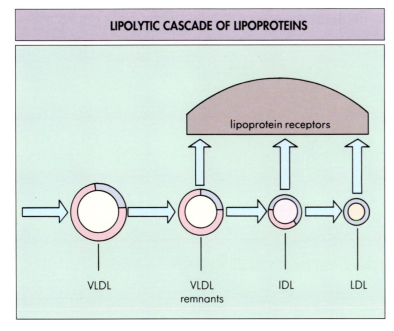

Fig. 1.24 The breakdown of triglyceride-rich lipoproteins (VLDL) into IDL and LDL by the lipolytic cascade in plasma.

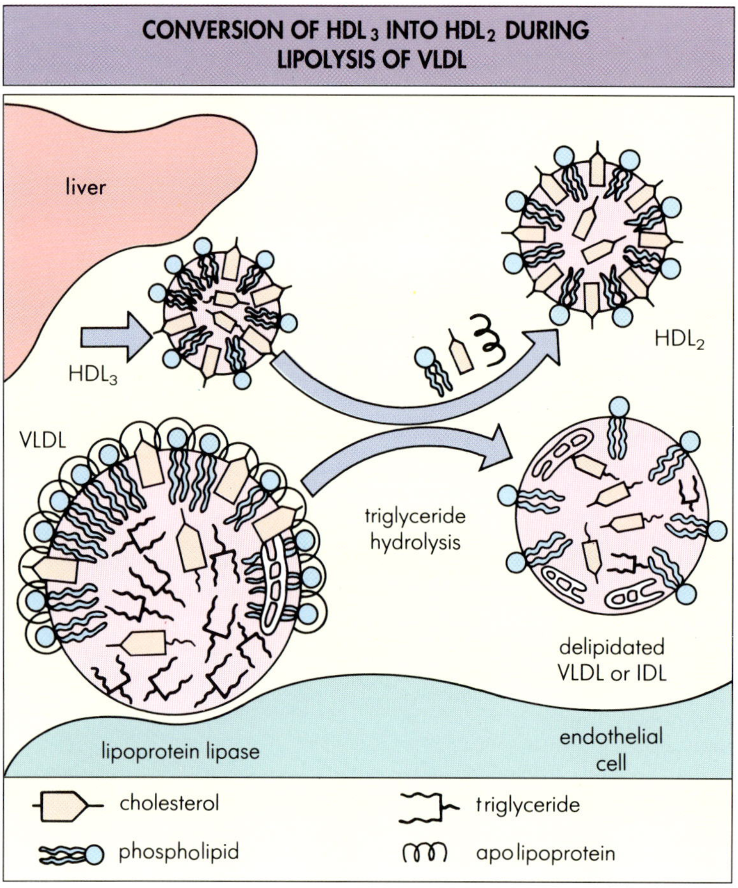

The Chemistry of Lipids

Fig. 1.25 Conversion of HDL_3 to HDL_2 through the incorporation of phospholipid, cholesterol, and proteins, released from VLDL during its lipolysis.

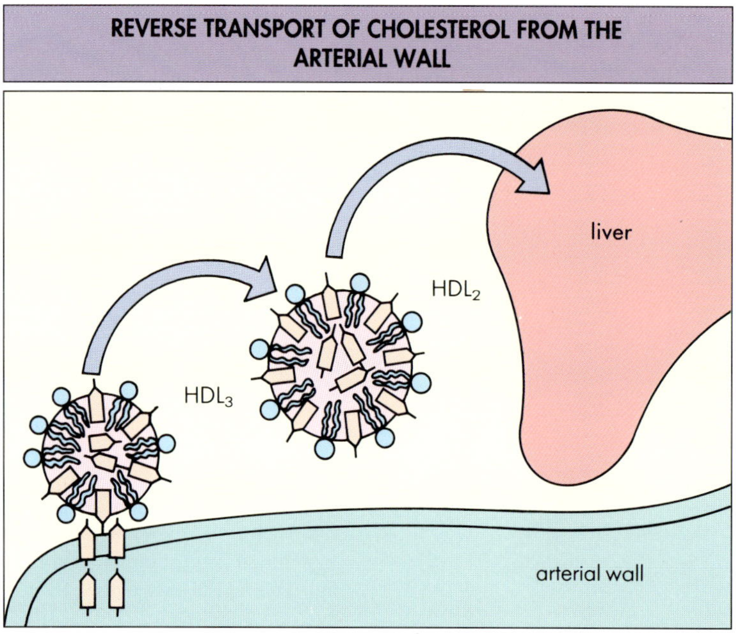

Fig. 1.26 A simplified scheme for the reverse transport of cholesterol from peripheral tissues such as the arterial wall, back to the liver.

SOURCES OF HIGH-DENSITY LIPOPROTEINS

Nascent HDL particles are secreted as disc-shaped structures by the liver and intestines. They are then modified in the plasma by association with other apolipoproteins and, particularly the enzyme, lecithin:cholesterol acyltransferase (LCAT), which converts them into spherical particles. They are further modified during the lipolytic breakdown of VLDL into IDL during which the small HDL_3 particle picks up surface components of VLDL, such as phospholipids and apolipoproteins C and E. The small HDL_3 particle transforms into the larger HDL_2 particle (Fig. 1.25). High-density lipoproteins may also be involved in the reverse transport of cholesterol from peripheral tissues such as the arterial wall, back to the liver for further metabolism, for example, into bile salts (Fig. 1.26). Cholesterol may be picked up by HDL_3 from the peripheral cell membrane, and converted to cholesteryl ester (by the action of LCAT), for transport in the core of the HDL particle to the liver. The body can deplete its peripheral stores of cholesterol and excrete it as bile salts into the intestines by this mechanism.

The circulation of lipoproteins

The circulation of endogenous (liver-derived) lipoproteins is shown in Fig. 1.27. The rate of output of liver VLDL depends on the rate of supply of free fatty acids from adipose-tissue stores and also on the rate of supply of glucose needed to synthesize glycerol. The pathway may be under regulation by insulin. Under conditions of caloric excess, the liver would be expected to synthesize and secrete large amounts of VLDL; however, even in the fasting state, the liver secretes VLDL from the influx of free fatty acids mobilized from adipose tissue, and this maintains the fasting levels of plasma triglycerides. A more detailed scheme for the circulation of both endogenous and exogenous lipoproteins is shown in Fig. 1.28. Many uncertainties, however, still exist in this scheme; for example, what quantities of IDL are removed directly by cell receptors or metabolized to LDL; or how many chylomicrons are metabolized to LDL or removed directly by remnant receptors?

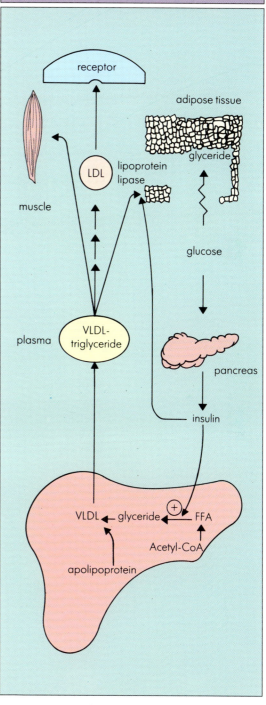

Fig. 1.27 A simplified scheme for the circulation and breakdown of triglyceride-rich lipoproteins secreted from the liver. FFA = free fatty acids.

The Chemistry of Lipids

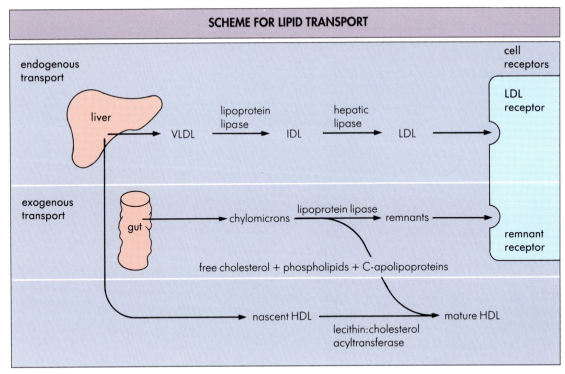

Fig. 1.28 A detailed scheme for the endogenous (liver) or exogenous (gut) transport of blood fats with some of the enzymes and regulatory proteins.

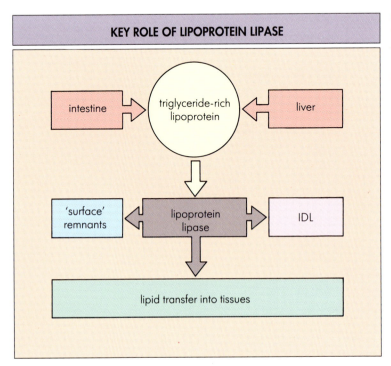

Fig. 1.29 The role of lipoprotein lipase in lipid transport and in the conversion of triglyceride-rich lipoproteins into other denser lipoproteins.

Enzymes involved in lipid transport

Lipoprotein lipase

Lipoprotein lipase determines the rate of removal of hepatic and intestinal triglyceride-rich lipoproteins from the bloodstream (Fig. 1.29). It catalyzes the sequential hydrolysis of core triglyceride into di- and monoglycerides, and also the final breakdown to free fatty acids and glycerol for uptake by peripheral tissues (Fig. 1.30). The enzyme is synthesized in parenchymal cells, such as heart, muscle, and adipose tissue. It is subsequently secreted by these cells into the capillary system for attachment to the luminal surface of endothelial cells. There it binds circulating VLDL and chylomicrons for hydrolysis of their core lipid, requiring apolipoprotein CII as an activator (Fig. 1.31). Once chylomicrons attach to endothelial cells, the cells

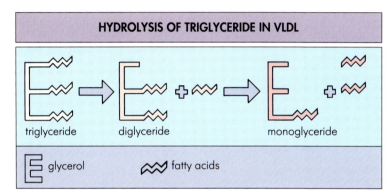

Fig. 1.30 A scheme for the breakdown of triglycerides in VLDL, by the action of lipoprotein lipase. Apolipoprotein CII increases, while apolipoprotein CIII may decrease the catalytic activity of lipoprotein lipase.

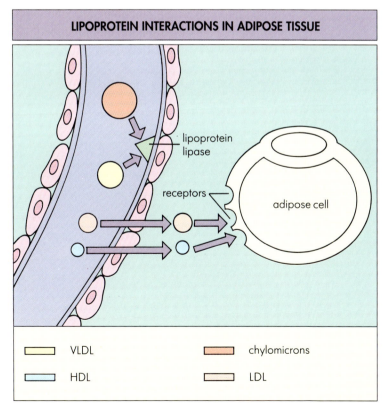

Fig. 1.31 Lipoprotein interactions in adipose tissue. The site of action of lipoprotein lipase is on the capillary endothelial cell where it binds to, and hyrolyses, chylomicrons or VLDL. The enzyme is secreted by parenchymal cells.

fill up with vacuoles containing fats derived from circulating lipoproteins (Fig. 1.32). The particles are sequentially delipidated and eventually converted into the cholesterol-rich particle, LDL. Under fed conditions, lipoprotein lipase is induced in adipose tissue where it diverts dietary fat for storage. Under fasting conditions, the enzyme level decreases in the capillary bed of adipose tissue, and the enzyme is induced in muscle and heart to divert VLDL to these sites for uptake of fatty acids as an additional fuel supply to glucose.

During lactation, there is a great increase in the levels of lipoprotein lipase in the capillary bed of the mammary gland, and blood fat is diverted into the secreted milk.

Hepatic lipase

Hepatic lipase is similar to lipoprotein lipase except it is only made in the liver and does not require apolipoprotein CII as an activator. It is also involved in the sequential lipolytic breakdown of triglyceride-rich lipoproteins, particularly IDL and remnant particles.

Lecithin:cholesterol acyltransferase

Lecithin:cholesterol acyltransferase esterifies the reactive hydroxyl group of cholesterol with a fatty acid derived from lecithin, thus converting cholesterol into a more apolar molecule for transport in the core, rather than in the shell of the lipoprotein particle (Fig. 1.33). The enzyme is used in the maturation of nascent HDL secreted by the liver, and also possibly in the reverse transport of cholesterol from peripheral tissues by HDL, back to the liver. Defects in this enzyme can occur, although very rarely, resulting in, for example, an accumulation of cholesterol and lipids in the cornea, thus producing a dense opacity (Fig. 1.34).

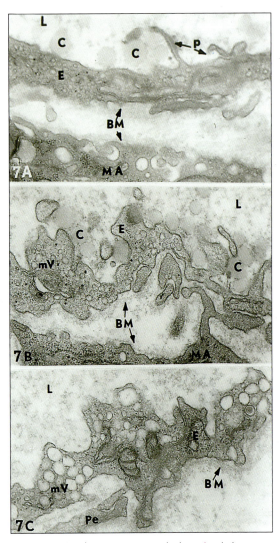

Fig. 1.32 An electron micrograph showing chylomicrons (C) binding to the endothelial lining (E) of capillaries which during hydrolysis fill up with fat vacuoles. L = lumen; BM = basement membrane.

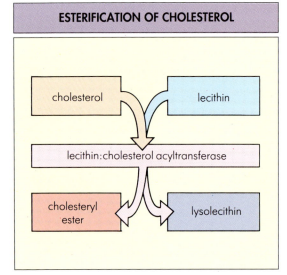

Fig. 1.33 Esterification of cholesterol catalyzed by lecithin:cholesterol acyltransferase. The enzyme is used in the modification of the HDL particle, apolipoprotein AI being a cofactor.

Lipids as Fuels: Transport

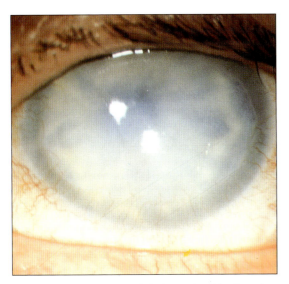

Fig. 1.34 Accumulation of cholesterol and lipids in the cornea, producing a dense opacity, can be due to a defect in lecithin:cholesterol acyltransferase.

Cholesteryl-ester transfer protein

Other proteins, such as the cholesteryl-ester transfer protein (CETP), are involved in the exchange of cholesteryl esters amongst the different lipoproteins and between peripheral cells and lipoproteins. Mutants of these proteins have been found, but do not appear to be associated with premature atherosclerosis.

Receptors involved in lipoprotein catabolism

Low-density lipoprotein receptor

The delipidation of VLDL leads to LDL which delivers cholesterol to peripheral cells. The LDL particle binds to special LDL receptors found as clusters in the coated pits of the cell membrane (Fig. 1.35). The LDL-receptor complex enters the cell as an endosome. The receptor is split off and possibly recycled back to the cell membrane. The endosome is acidified and converts to a lysosome. The apolipoprotein-B peptide is digested by lysosomal enzymes, and the cholesterol is liberated for use by the cell in the manufacture of cell membranes. At the same time, intracellular cholesterol synthesis is switched off by inhibiting the key enzyme, HMGCoA reductase.

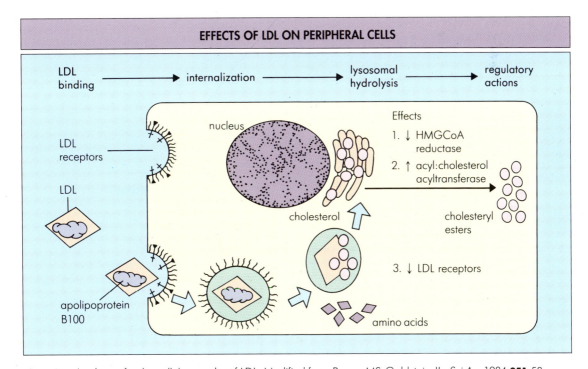

Fig. 1.35 A scheme for the cellular uptake of LDL. Modified from Brown MS, Goldstein JL. *Sci Am* 1984;**251**:58.

The structure of the LDL receptor was determined by Brown and Goldstein (Nobel Laureates for Medicine in 1985) (Fig. 1.36). The receptor is divided into functional parts or domains, some of the key elements being the binding domain for LDL (the ligand), the membrane-spanning domain which anchors the receptor into the cell membrane, and the intracellular portion of the molecule which is involved in the formation of endosomes. Mutations at any of these sites can interfere with the function of the receptor, such as migration to coated pits, or attachment to the cell membrane, leading to the disease, Familial Hypercholesterolaemia. The complicated regulation of the LDL receptor underlines the importance of proper homeostatic mechanisms in the body in order to maintain physiological pools of cholesterol and to prevent overloading of peripheral tissue sites.

Remnant receptor

During the circulation of lipoproteins (see *Fig. 1.28*), chylomicron remnants are believed to be removed by an additional receptor, the remnant receptor. A possible candidate, which bears some resemblance to the LDL receptor, has recently been discovered (Fig. 1.37). However, work is still required in this area to prove whether this is in fact the receptor involved in the removal of remnants.

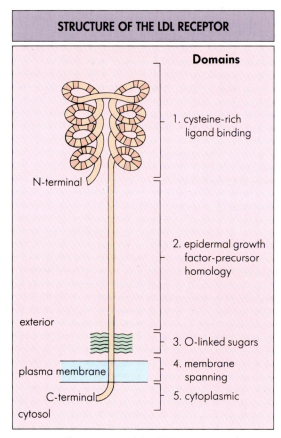

Fig. 1.36 The structure of the LDL receptor can be divided into domains subserving separate functions. The head of the molecule binds to apolipoprotein B100 of the LDL particle and initiates the uptake of the particle into the cell. Modified from Brown MS, Goldstein JL. *Sci Am* 1984;**251**:58.

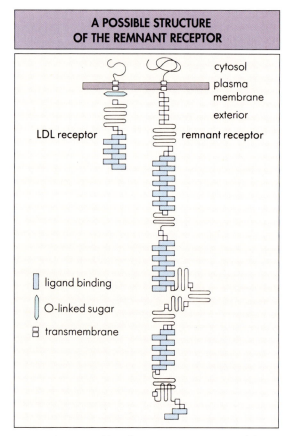

Fig. 1.37 A possible schematic representation of the remnant receptor which may remove chylomicron remnants. The receptor bears some resemblance to the LDL receptor.

DETERMINATION OF THE LEVELS OF CHOLESTEROL AND TRIGLYCERIDE

Enzymatic assays

The older colorimetric assays which were used to determine concentrations of cholesterol and triglycerides have been superseded by specific enzymatic assays that involve linked enzyme reactions. Assays for measuring both cholesterol (Fig. 1.38) and triglyceride concentrations (Fig. 1.39) yield H_2O_2 which reacts with a chromogen to produce a coloured product that can be read in a spectrophotometer at an absorbance of A520. Since the same coloured chromogen is produced in both the triglyceride and cholesterol assays, the same settings of the spectrophotometer can be used. A simple flow sheet for the discrete analyser is shown in Fig. 1.40. In order to ensure accuracy and reproducibility of the assays, standard sera should be used, and different laboratories can exchange samples to ensure quality control.

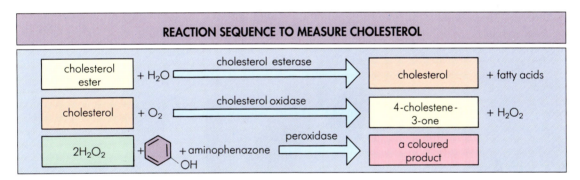

Fig. 1.38 A scheme for the estimation of plasma cholesterol using enzymatic reactions involving cholesterol oxidase.

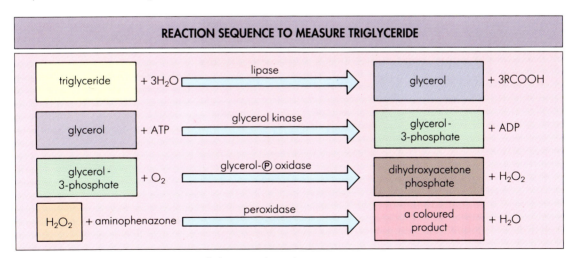

Fig. 1.39 A scheme for the estimation of plasma triglyceride using enzymatic reactions involving lipases.

The Chemistry of Lipids

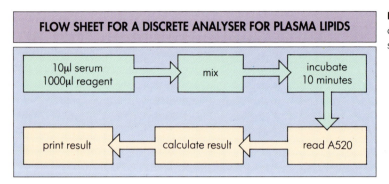

Fig. 1.40 A flow sheet for a discrete analyser to measure the levels of serum cholesterol and triglyceride.

The Reflotron

Recently, instruments such as the Reflotron have been designed to measure cholesterol or triglyceride concentrations in a drop of blood in the doctor's surgery or out-patient clinic, with the results being available within 2–3 minutes (Fig. 1.41). The Reflotron is very similar to glucometers which are used to monitor the treatment of diabetics by measuring the blood glucose concentrations in drops of capillary blood. Immediate availability of plasma cholesterol and triglyceride results is of great help in the management of hyperlipidaemia since it can encourage patient compliance to diets and drugs. Many other instruments which use 'dry' chemistry on paper strips to measure blood cholesterol and triglyceride, are also now available (Fig. 1.42).

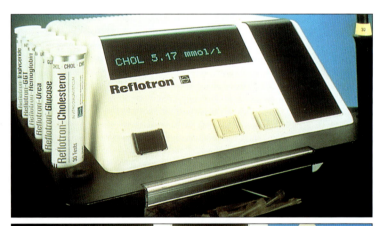
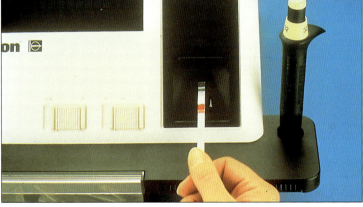

Fig. 1.41 Reflotron instrument used to measure the levels of cholesterol and triglyceride in a finger prick of whole blood.

Determination of the Levels of Cholesterol and Triglyceride

INSTRUMENTS AVAILABLE TO MEASURE LEVELS OF CHOLESTEROL AND TRIGLYCERIDES	
Group 1	
Reflotron	Boehringer Mannheim UK (Diagnostics and Biochemicals Ltd) Bell Lane Lewes East Sussex, BM7 1LG
Vision	Abbott Diagnostics Division Abbott House Moorbridge Road Maidenhead Berkshire, SL6 8XZ
Group 2	
Kodak DT60	Kodak Ltd PO Box 66 Station Road Hemel Hempstead Herts, HP1 1JU
Ames Seralyzer	Ames Division Miles Ltd Stoke Court Stoke Poges Slough, SL2 4LY
Analyst	DuPont Diagnostics Division Dupont UK Ltd Wedgewood Way Stevenage Herts, SU1 4QN
Easy ST	Olympus Biomedical Products Division Olympus House 7 West Links Tollgate Eastleigh Hampshire, SO5 3TP

Fig. 1.42 Other instruments available to measure the levels of cholesterol and triglyceride in the out-patient clinic.

CHAPTER TWO

Inherited Defects of Lipid Metabolism

The subject of inherited defects of carbohydrate and lipid metabolism was founded by Sir Archibald Garrod (1857–1936), a physician at St Bartholomew's Hospital, London (Fig. 2.1). He postulated that abnormal genes can produce abnormal enzymes or proteins, thus leading to a metabolic disease (Fig. 2.2). He initially studied disorders, such as alkaptonuria, pentosuria, and albinism, but his ideas have extended to all other metabolic diseases which have a genetic basis. The most common defects in lipid metabolism are those of transport which give rise to hyperlipidaemia, and those of storage which cause, most importantly, premature atherosclerosis.

DISORDERS OF LIPID TRANSPORT: THE HYPERLIPIDAEMIAS

There are five main disorders of lipid transport that were initially classified by Fredrickson (Fig. 2.3) according to the lipoprotein which accumulates in plasma samples (Fig. 2.4), and diagnosis in

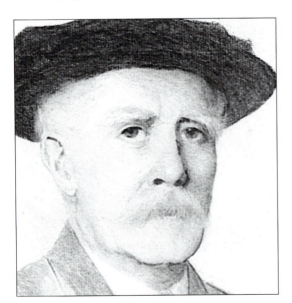

Fig. 2.1 Sir Archibald Garrod (aged 65), founding father of inherited defects of metabolism.

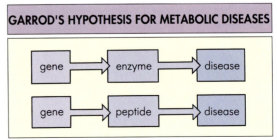

Fig. 2.2 Garrod's hypothesis for the origin of inherited metabolic diseases.

Disorders of Lipid Transport: The Hyperlipidaemias

THE FREDRICKSON CLASSIFICATION OF THE HYPERLIPIDAEMIAS				
Type of hyperlipidaemia	Lipoprotein accumulation	Lipid accumulation	Biochemical lesion	Some clinical features

I	chylomicrons	triglyceride	defect of lipoprotein lipase
			
			defect of apolipoprotein CII
				Familial
				  rare
				  acute abdominal pain
				  pancreatitis
				  eruptive xanthomata
				  lipaemia retinalis
				  diagnosis in childhood
				Secondary
				  dysgammaglobulinaemia

IIa	LDL	cholesterol	Monogenic
			  impaired receptor for LDL catabolism
			
			  mutants of apolipoprotein B100
			Polygenic
			  possibly LDL receptor
				Familial
				  common (1:500)
				  dominant inheritance
				  tendon xanthomata
				Secondary
				  nephrotic syndrome
				  hypothyroidism
				  dysgammaglobulinaemia

IIb	LDL VLDL	cholesterol triglyceride	gene defects unknown	xanthomata early atheroma

III	abnormal lipoprotein migrating ahead of β–lipoprotein (IDL)	cholesterol
		triglyceride
			defect of conversion of VLDL to LDL	Familial Dysbetalipoproteinaemia
				  rare
				  recessive
				  palmar xanthomata

IV	VLDL	triglyceride
		cholesterol
			increased triglyceride synthesis; defect in peripheral clearance (as possible abnormalities)	Primary
				  cutaneous xanthomata
				Secondary
				  diabetes
				  alcoholism
				  obesity
				  pregnancy
				  oestrogen therapy
				  hypothyroidism
				  steroid therapy

V	chylomicrons
	VLDL
		triglyceride
		cholesterol
			similar mechanisms to Type IV	Primary
				  rare
				  cutaneous xanthomata
				Secondary
				  diabetes
				  alcoholism

All the above hyperlipidaemias, with the exception of Type I, may predispose to degenerative arterial disease.				

Fig. 2.3 The Fredrickson classification of the hyperlipidaemias.

Inherited Defects of Lipid Metabolism

some cases can be made by carrying out a simple visual inspection of a fasting plasma sample in a test tube. Type I or Type V hyperlipidaemias can be identified by the presence of a creamy layer that floats to the top of the tube, which has either a clear or turbid infranatant. An alternative classification based on aetiology is also useful for clinicians to clarify treatment of the possible causes.

A simple way to consider the origin of the hyperlipidaemias is to use the pool concept of input and output of lipids from the plasma compartment (Fig. 2.5): an increased inflow of triglyceride from the liver, or a decreased output into peripheral tissues, will result in hypertriglyceridaemia, and similarly for hypercholesterolaemia.

Causes of the inflow–outflow defects can be primarily genetic or environmental (with a genetic predisposition). The acquired causes are often due to other systemic diseases, such as hypothyroidism or diabetes mellitus. The clinical classification of hyperlipidaemias which is referred to in this book, is presented in Fig. 2.6. On this basis, Familial Hypercholesterolaemia is defined as a monogenic disorder of LDL outflow from the plasma due to a defect in the LDL receptor, and Familial Combined Hyperlipidaemia is defined as a polygenic disorder (the genetic basis has not yet been elucidated) which gives rise to an elevation of levels of plasma LDL and/or VLDL. The common hyperlipidaemias are now considered.

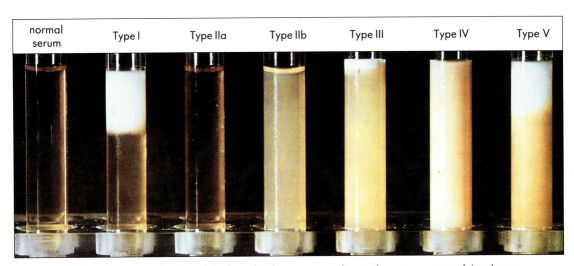

Fig. 2.4 The Fredrickson classification of the hyperlipidaemias according to the appearances of the plasma.

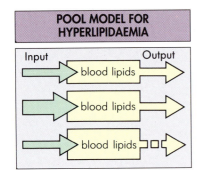

Fig. 2.5 The pool concept for hyperlipidaemia. The thick arrow indicates increased flow and the dotted arrow indicates decreased outflow from the blood compartment.

CLINICAL CLASSIFICATION OF THE HYPERLIPIDAEMIAS

Disease	Elevation of plasma	
	Cholesterol	Triglyceride

Familial or Primary	Familial Hypercholesterolaemia
	i. monogenic
	   LDL-receptor defects
	   B-100 defects
	ii. polygenic
		Familial Hypertriglyceridaemia
		i. monogenic
		   lipase defect
		   apolipoprotein-CII defect
		ii. polygenic
		   Familial combined

Secondary	hypothyroidism nephrotic syndrome diabetes mellitus biliary cirrhosis	diabetes mellitus alcoholism obesity carbohydrate induced

Fig. 2.6 A clinical classification of the hyperlipidaemias.

Disorders of Lipid Transport: The Hyperlipidaemias

Familial or Primary Hypertriglyceridaemia: Fredrickson Type I

Defects of lipoprotein lipase

This type of Familial Hypertriglyceridaemia is a rare, autosomal recessive disorder in which there is a defect of the enzyme, lipoprotein lipase, thus impairing clearance of VLDL and/or chylomicrons from the plasma. Very rarely, this disorder can occur secondary to a dysgammaglobulinaemia which interferes with the function of lipoprotein lipase.

The condition appears in childhood or adult life and involves episodes of acute abdominal pain (due to acute pancreatitis), eruptive xanthomata (Fig. 2.7), and lipaemia retinalis (Fig. 2.8). Once suspected clinically, the diagnosis is established by the appearance of the plasma, and by measuring the level of lipids (Fig. 2.9). Measurements of the activity of lipoprotein lipase in adipose tissue or muscle, define the nature of the defect.

The main aim of treatment is to reduce the level of fats in the blood as quickly as possible by diet and drugs (fibrates or nicotinates), thus preventing further attacks of acute pancreatitis or retinal vascular thrombosis (see *Chapter 9*). Reduction of long-chain triglycerides in the diet to less than 15g/day, and substitution with short- or medium-chain triglycerides (making a total daily intake of less than 25g/day) will reduce the chylomicron-aemia. The fatty acids of short- or medium-chain

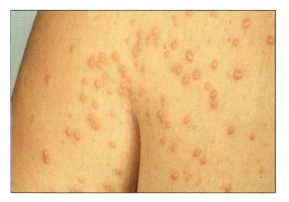

Fig. 2.7 Crops of eruptive xanthomata appearing over the skin of a patient with Familial Hyperlipidaemia. The histology of these lesions resembles the fatty streak of the arterial wall.

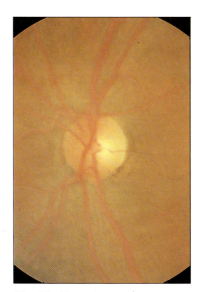

Fig. 2.8 Lipaemia retinalis in a patient with Familial Hypertriglycerid-aemia, Fredrickson Type I. Note the milky-white appearance of the retinal blood vessels due to dilution with fat-containing particles.

PLASMA FEATURES OF TYPE 1 HYPERLIPIDAEMIA

Lipoprotein phenotype	Plasma cholesterol	Plasma triglyceride	Plasma appearance
Type I — chylomicrons ↑↑↑	normal to moderately elevated	markedly elevated	'cream layer' above clear to slightly turbid infranatant

Fig. 2.9 Characteristic plasma features of Familial Hypertriglyceridaemia, Fredrickson Type I.

Inherited Defects of Lipid Metabolism

triglycerides are absorbed directly into the portal vein and are not converted into chylomicrons by the intestine. Life-long adherence to this diet may be required.

The condition is not characteristically associated with premature atherosclerosis. Chylomicrons may not be atherogenic since their size excludes them from possible entry into the subendothelial space of the arterial wall, although chylomicron remnants may transport cholesteryl esters into the arterial wall for transfer by the action of cholesteryl-ester transfer protein (CETP).

Deficiency of apolipoprotein CII

Deficiency of apolipoprotein CII is a rare, autosomal recessive disorder where apolipoprotein CII is absent or defective. A failure to activate the enzyme, lipoprotein lipase, results in a clearance defect of triglyceride-rich lipoproteins. The disorder can also occur secondary to a dysgammaglobulinaemia that binds apolipoprotein CII, hence preventing the activation of lipoprotein lipase. The diagnostic and clinical features are very similar to those of familial lipoprotein-lipase deficiency.

CASE REPORTS

Case 1

A woman, aged 52 (Fig. 2.10), presented with episodes of acute abdominal pain since childhood. She had been admitted to hospital as often as four times a year because of acute pancreatitis. She presented with small eruptive xanthomata, splenomegaly that was probably due to fat infiltration, and lipaemia retinalis. Her fasting plasma indicated chylomicronaemia (Fig. 2.11), plasma triglycerides were 24mM (2,124mg/dl), and her blood monocytes were transformed into foam cells (cells filled with lipid vacuoles) (Fig. 2.12). Biopsy of her adipose tissue revealed no measurable activity of lipoprotein lipase (Fig. 2.13), thus establishing the diagnosis of Familial Hypertriglyceridaemia. She was treated with drugs and low-fat diets which required substitution of long-chain triglycerides with medium-chain triglycerides. One of her brothers also had hypertriglyceridaemia.

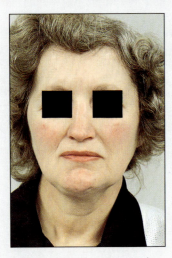

Fig. 2.10 A woman, aged 52, with Familial Hypertriglyceridaemia, Fredrickson Type I, due to a defect of lipoprotein lipase.

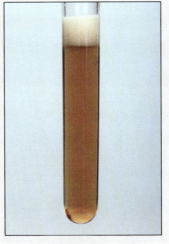

Fig. 2.11 A fasting plasma sample of the patient, showing the chylomicron layer at the top of the tube with a turbid infranatant.

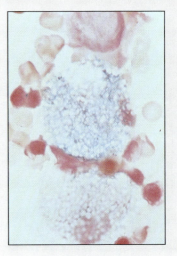

Fig. 2.12 White blood cells showing gross fat accumulation in the patient.

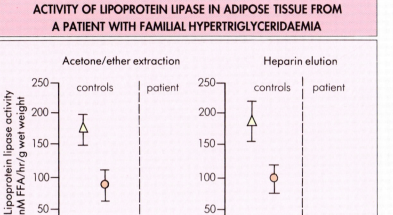

Fig. 2.13 The activity of lipoprotein lipase in adipose tissue in the patient compared to that in normotriglyceridaemic controls. No detectable enzyme activity can be seen in the patient. Data modified from Durrington PN, Holdsworth G, Galton DJ. *Ann Int Med* 1981;**94**:211.

Case 2

A man, aged 53 (Fig. 2.14), was found to have fasting chylomicronaemia (Fig. 2.15), lipaemia retinalis, severe Raynaud's phenomenon, and white blood cells which showed early accumulation of triglyceride vacuoles (Fig. 2.16). Gel electrophoresis of his

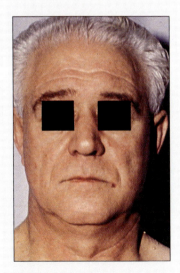

Fig. 2.14 A man, aged 53, with a deficiency of apolipoprotein CII.

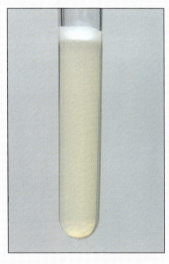

Fig. 2.15 A fasting plasma sample of the patient, showing chylomicronaemia.

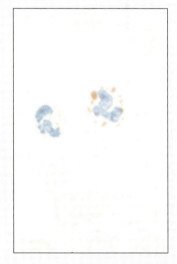

Fig. 2.16 White blood cells showing early accumulation of triglyceride vacuoles.

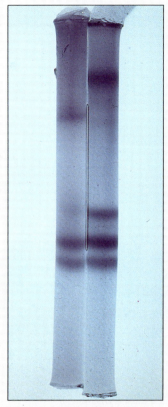

Fig. 2.17 Gel electrophoresis of the C-apolipoproteins from the patient (left-hand track) and a control (right-hand track). The patient shows a missing upper band which is apolipoprotein CII.

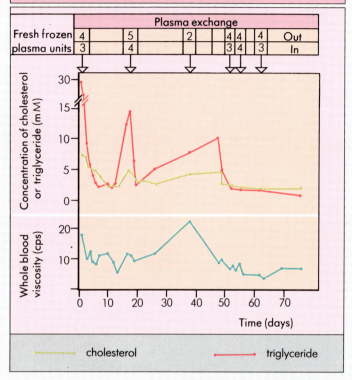

Fig. 2.18 Changes in levels of plasma triglyceride and cholesterol of the patient with apolipoprotein-CII deficiency who was infused with fresh frozen plasma. Data modified from Reckless JPD, Stocks J, Galton DJ, Suggett B, Walton K. *Clin Sci* 1982;**62**:93.

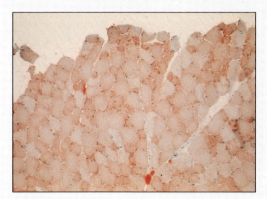

Fig. 2.19 A muscle biopsy showing abnormal accumulation of triglycerides which are stained with oil-red O.

C-apolipoproteins showed an almost complete absence of the CII peptide (Fig. 2.17). After transfusion with three units of fresh frozen plasma, the concentration of plasma apolipoprotein CII was restored to normal, and levels of plasma triglycerides fell precipitately from 30mM (2655mg/dl) to 2.5mM (221mg/dl) (Fig. 2.18). Levels of plasma triglyceride again increased over the following 10 days: this increase, however, responded dramatically to a further infusion of four units of fresh frozen plasma. An accumulation of triglycerides in his muscles also occurred (Fig. 2.19). Long-term treatment for this condition is the same as for disorders of lipoprotein lipase.

Disorders of Lipid Transport: The Hyperlipidaemias

Other abnormalities of apolipoprotein CII

Other disorders of the production of apolipoprotein CII may occur which interfere with the substrate properties of VLDL for the catalytic activity of lipoprotein lipase.

CASE REPORT

A boy, aged 13 (Fig. 2.20), was found to have severe chylomicronaemia and lipaemia retinalis. Gel electrophoresis of his C-apolipoproteins showed a relative increase in the concentration of apolipoprotein CII compared to apolipoprotein CIII (Fig. 2.21). By measuring the direct release of fatty acids from his lipoproteins, chylomicrons were found to be inefficient substrates for lipoprotein lipase and were found to carry excess apolipoprotein CII. It is most likely that the proportions of apolipoproteins need to be kept within strictly defined limits in order to allow for their optimal breakdown by lipoprotein lipase and satisfactory clearance from the plasma compartment. He was commenced on low-fat diets and fibrates, which brought his lipid levels towards the normal range.

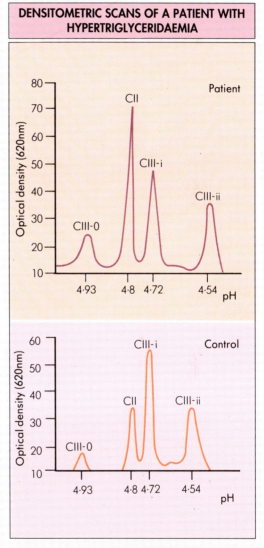

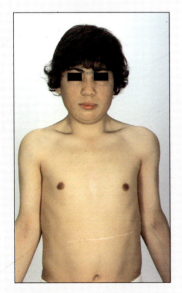

Fig. 2.20 A young boy, aged 13, who presented with fasting chylomicronaemia.

Fig. 2.21 Gel electrophoresis of C-apolipoproteins. Lower panel: The normal proportions of C-apolipoproteins in triglyceride-rich lipoproteins. Upper panel: Concentration of the C-apolipoproteins in the patient. Note a relative increase in the concentration of apolipoprotein CII compared to apolipoprotein CIII. Data modified from Stocks J, Holdsworth G, Dodson PM, Galton DJ. *Atherosclerosis* 1981;**38**:1.

Inherited Defects of Lipid Metabolism

Familial Hypertriglyceridaemia: Fredrickson Type IV

Polygenic Familial Hypertriglyceridaemia

Polygenic Familial Hypertriglyceridaemia is a common heterogeneous group of disorders in which a genetic predisposition interacts with environmental factors such as dietary intake of fat or carbohydrate, to produce hypertriglyceridaemia; the diagnostic features are presented in Fig. 2.22. Possible causative factors are an increased synthesis of VLDL by the liver and/or an impaired clearance of VLDL by peripheral tissues. This type of hyperlipidaemia can cause ectopic lipid deposition at the corneal–scleral junction (Fig. 2.23) and eruptive xanthomata over the skin (Fig. 2.24). The condition is probably atherogenic and should be actively treated. The principal guidelines for treatment are reduction of body weight, and reduction of animal fats in the diet. If levels of plasma triglyceride fail to respond to simple dietary measures, hypolipidaemic drugs such as fibrates, nicotinates, or marine oils, should be administered (see *Chapter 9*).

PLASMA FEATURES OF TYPE IV HYPERLIPIDAEMIA

Lipoprotein phenotype	Plasma cholesterol	Plasma triglyceride	Plasma appearance
Type IV — VLDL ↑↑↑	normal to slightly elevated	moderately to markedly elevated	turbid to frankly opaque

Fig. 2.22 Characteristic plasma features of polygenic Familial Hypertriglyceridaemia, Fredrickson Type IV.

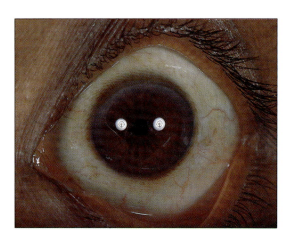

Fig. 2.23 A patient with polygenic hypertriglyceridaemia. On close inspection, a milky-white arcus is observed that is quite different from the 'hard' cholesterol arcus of Familial Hypercholesterolaemia.

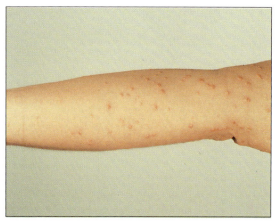

Fig. 2.24 Crops of eruptive xanthomata in a patient with polygenic hypertriglyceridaemia.

CASE REPORT

A man, aged 46 (member 1 in Fig. 2.25), presented with a left-branch retinal-vein occlusion which resulted in blurred vision. Although he was not hypertensive or diabetic, three samples of fasting lipid revealed serum triglyceride levels of 6.1, 8.0, and 6.1mM (540, 708, and 540mg/dl) and serum cholesterol levels of 5.2, 5.8, and 5.6mM (201, 224, and 217mg/dl). He consumed approximately six units of alcohol at weekends only, and his gammaglutamyl transferase levels were normal at 13u/l. No symptoms of arterial disease were present, but his exercise ECG showed mild ST depression in leads 2, 3, aVF, and V5–6, after one minute. Family screening revealed that his daughter, aged 11 years, had a raised fasting plasma triglyceride level of 4.9mM (434mg/dl), and his son also had elevated lipid levels (Fig. 2.25). All three were treated by dietary reduction of animal fats, which successfully brought the plasma lipids to within the normal range. There has been no recurrence of retinal vascular thrombosis in the father. A possible genetic component in this family was shown by the inheritance of an allele of apolipoprotein AI in the affected members, which was not found in the unaffected mother and daughter (Fig. 2.25).

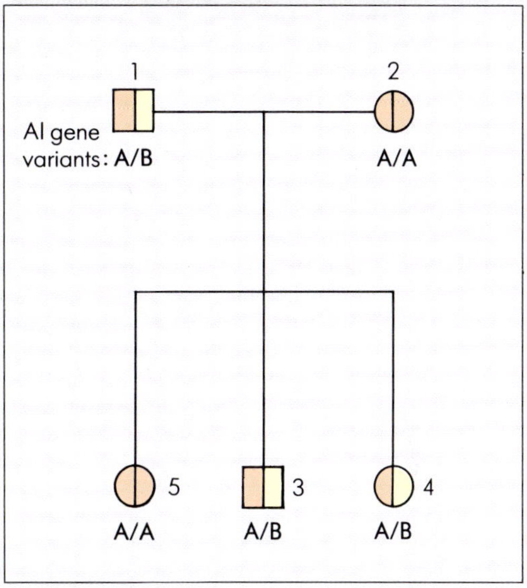

Fig. 2.25 Pedigree with polygenic Familial Hypertriglyceridaemia, Fredrickson Type IV, showing the inheritance of an allele of apolipoprotein AI (A or B) and hypertriglyceridaemia. The proband (1) is hypertriglyceridaemic and the mother (2) is normolipidaemic. The children (3) aged 12 years and (4) 11 years had triglyceride values above normal for their age. The child (5) aged 18 years was normolipidaemic. Modified from Rees A, Stocks J, Sharpe CR et al. *J Clin Invest* 1985;**76**:1090.

Severe hypertriglyceridaemia (Chylomicronaemia syndrome): Fredrickson Type V

Severe hypertriglyceridaemia forms a spectrum with the polygenic hypertriglyceridaemias, and is characterized by a gross accumulation of triglyceride-rich lipoproteins (both VLDL and chylomicrons) in plasma. Uncontrolled diabetes mellitus is often the precipitating environmental factor in an individual who is already predisposed to develop hypertriglyceridaemia. The characteristic plasma features of this disorder are presented in Fig. 2.26, and diagnostic features include:
- profuse eruptive xanthomata
- recurrent bouts of acute pancreatitis
- lipaemia retinalis
- retinal vascular occlusions

The main guidelines for treatment are to bring the secondary conditions (such as diabetes mellitus) under control, commence a low animal-fat diet (less than 15g/day), use hypolipidaemic drugs (fibrates or nicotinates), and in severe cases, perform plasma exchange.

Inherited Defects of Lipid Metabolism

PLASMA FEATURES OF TYPE V HYPERLIPIDAEMIA			
Lipoprotein phenotype	Plasma cholesterol	Plasma triglyceride	Plasma appearance
Type V chylomicrons ↑↑↑ VLDL ↑↑	moderately elevated	markedly elevated	'cream layer' over turbid to opaque infranatant

Fig. 2.26 Characteristic plasma features of severe hypertriglyceridaemia, Fredrickson Type V.

CASE REPORT

A woman, aged 37 (Fig. 2.27), presented with widespread eruptive xanthomata and bouts of acute pancreatitis. She suffered from diabetes mellitus which was very poorly controlled, and she refused to take her full dosage of insulin. The appearances of her plasma are shown in Fig. 2.28. Two litres of her plasma were exchanged with fresh frozen plasma (Fig. 2.29), resulting in the correction of her blood abnormalities (Fig. 2.30). Her lipid levels almost returned to normal, and her plasma viscosity was reduced to within the normal range. Her lipid levels should remain normal with the institution of proper diabetic and dietary therapy.

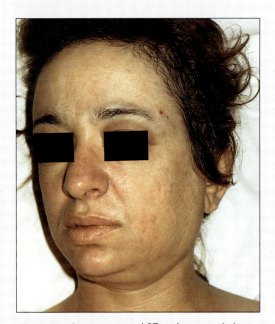

Fig. 2.27 A woman, aged 37, with severe diabetic hypertriglyceridaemia, Fredrickson Type V.

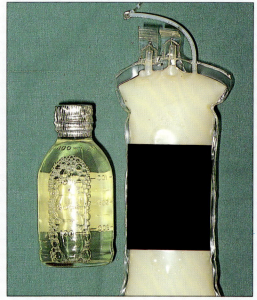

Fig. 2.28 Turbid plasma from the patient, removed during exchange transfusion.

Disorders of Lipid Transport: The Hyperlipidaemias

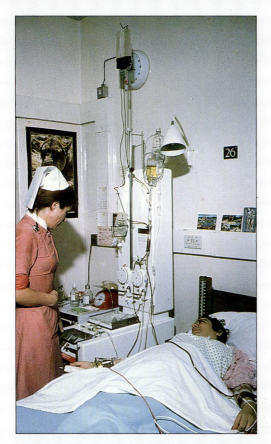

Fig. 2.29 Plasma exchange being carried out to lower the blood lipids of the patient. The cell separator is by the right-hand side of the bed.

Fig. 2.30 Correction of blood abnormalities after plasma exchange. Data modified from Betteridge DJ, Taylor KM, Reckless JPD, de Silva R, Galton DJ. *Lancet* 1978;**i**:1368.

Familial Dyslipoproteinaemia/ 'Broad-beta' disease: Fredrickson Type III

Familial Dyslipoproteinaemia is a polygenic disorder in which an abnormal IDL accumulates in the plasma due to a defect in the VLDL lipolytic cascade. As a result, a 'broad-beta' lipoprotein accumulates, which carries roughly equal amounts of cholesterol and triglyceride. Diagnostic features of this disorder include:
- Tuberous (Fig. 2.31) and planar (Fig. 2.32) xanthomata, particularly in the skin creases of the hands.
- A broad beta-migrating band on electrophoresis (Fig. 2.33).
- A 'floating' LDL-like band on ultracentrifugation. This band floats because of its triglyceride content (Fig. 2.34).
- 95% of cases have an E2 polymorphic apolipoprotein.

Since this hyperlipidaemia is very atherogenic, it is important to treat the condition promptly. Most cases respond well to diet and the administration of fibrates.

Inherited Defects of Lipid Metabolism

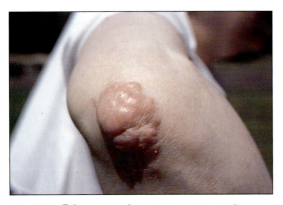

Fig. 2.31 Tuberous xanthomata in a patient with 'broad-beta' disease, Fredrickson Type III.

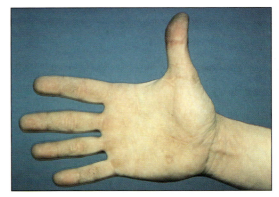

Fig. 2.32 Planar xanthomata in a patient with 'broad-beta' disease, Fredrickson Type III, showing the streaky deposits in the skin creases.

PLASMA FEATURES OF TYPE III HYPERLIPIDAEMIA

Lipoprotein phenotype	Plasma cholesterol	Plasma triglyceride	Plasma appearance
Type III — β-VLDL/LDL of abnormal composition	elevated	moderately to markedly elevated	turbid to frankly opaque 'cream layer' above turbid infranatant occasionally present

Fig. 2.33 Characteristic plasma features of Familial Dyslipoproteinaemia or 'broad-beta' disease, Fredrickson Type III. Note the βVLDL/LDL of abnormal composition.

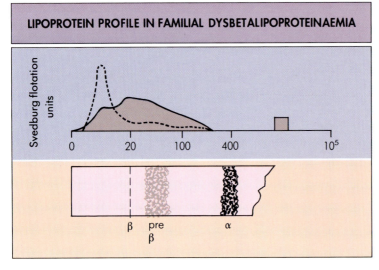

Fig. 2.34 The plasma lipoprotein pattern in Familial Dyslipoproteinaemia, Type III. Upper panel: Ultracentrifugal pattern of plasma lipoproteins run at a density of 1.063g/ml. The dotted line indicates normal plasma. The coloured area shows abnormal 'broad-beta' lipoprotein. Lower panel: 'Broad-beta' band on electrophoresis.

Disorders of Lipid Transport: The Hyperlipidaemias

Familial Combined Hyperlipidaemia: Fredrickson Type IIb

Familial Combined Hyperlipidaemia is a fairly common hyperlipidaemia which occurs in up to 0.5% of the Caucasian population. Levels of plasma LDL and/or VLDL are elevated in many individuals of a pedigree. The characteristic features of the plasma are shown in Fig. 2.35, and a typical pedigree is presented in Fig. 2.36. The lipoprotein phenotypes can be variable in the same

PLASMA FEATURES OF TYPE IIb HYPERLIPIDAEMIA

Lipoprotein phenotype	Plasma cholesterol	Plasma triglyceride	Plasma appearance
Type IIb 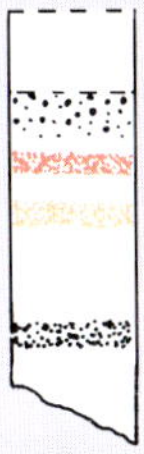 –LDL ↑↑↑ –VLDL ↑	elevated	moderately elevated	slightly to moderately turbid

Fig. 2.35 Characteristic plasma features of Familial Combined Hyperlipidaemia, Fredrickson Type IIb. Note the two heavy bands in the region of LDL and VLDL.

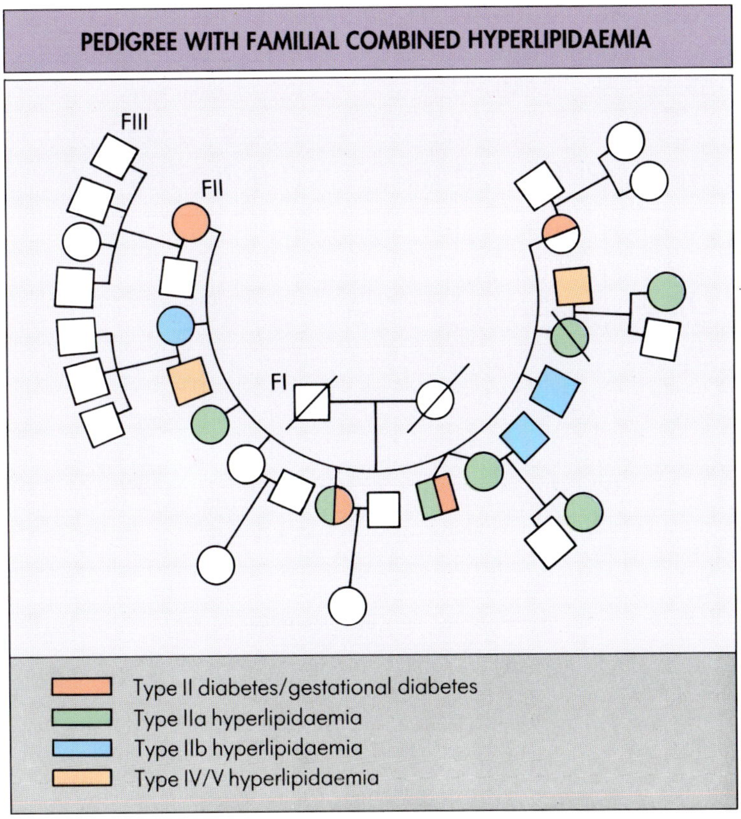

PEDIGREE WITH FAMILIAL COMBINED HYPERLIPIDAEMIA

- ■ Type II diabetes/gestational diabetes
- ■ Type IIa hyperlipidaemia
- ■ Type IIb hyperlipidaemia
- ■ Type IV/V hyperlipidaemia

Fig. 2.36 A pedigree in which Familial Combined Hyperlipidaemia, segregates. Note the varied types of hyperlipidaemia that occur in the family members.

individuals depending on their nutritional status. This condition has been found as the most common genetic form of hyperlipidaemia in relatives of survivors of myocardial infarction, occurring in up to 30% of the family members. The genetics of the condition, however, have not been elucidated; the condition may be due to either the variable expression of a single autosomal dominant gene, or to the co-segregation of two or more separate genes.

The condition is clearly atherogenic and should be treated actively on the following lines:

- reduction of body weight if obese
- low animal-fat/cholesterol diets
- administration of hypolipidaemic drugs (fibrates, nicotinates, statins)
- regular monitoring of plasma lipids to ensure benefits of therapy

Familial Hypercholesterolaemia: Fredrickson Type IIa

Familial Hypercholesterolaemia has been the most intensively studied hyperlipidaemia following the discovery of the LDL receptor which plays a major role in the removal of LDL-cholesterol from the blood. It is an autosomal dominant disorder occurring at a frequency of approximately 0.2% in Caucasian populations, and is due to a family of mutations occurring in the LDL-receptor gene on chromosome 19 (Fig. 2.37). These mutations involve deletions of part of the gene (for example, the French–Canadian mutation deletes exon 1 and regulatory sequences close to it), or point mutations which may alter the structure of the LDL-receptor protein and so interfere with LDL clearance from the blood. Other mutations are also described in Fig. 2.37. The presence of numerous DNA repeat sequences (called ALU repeats),

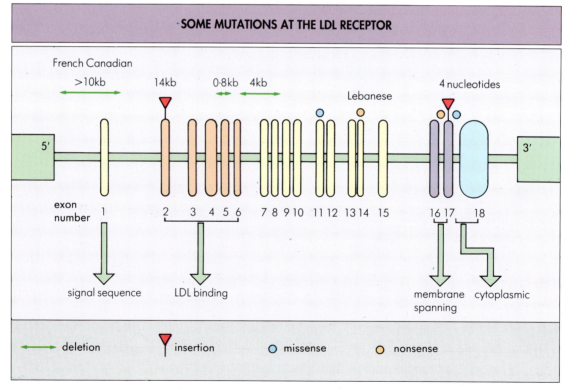

Fig. 2.37 Mutations in the LDL-receptor gene, resulting in Familial Hypercholesterolaemia, Fredrickson Type IIa. The major defects are deletions or insertions of DNA, point mutations which cause missense of the ensuing protein structure, or premature stop codons which terminate the protein sequence. Modified from Brown MS, Goldstein JL. *Atheroscl Rev* 1988;**18**:85.

Disorders of Lipid Transport: The Hyperlipidaemias

which makes unequal recombination between parental genes likely, may account for the many deletional mutants which occur in the LDL-receptor gene (Fig. 2.37).

Diagnosis of the disorder can be established by measurements of LDL-cholesterol in investigation of a plasma sample (Fig. 2.38), together with determination of the presence of ectopic cholesterol deposits in the cornea and extensor tendons of the hands or legs, and confirmation of a positive family history of early arterial disease.

Treatment is aimed at reducing the level of blood cholesterol to less than 6.5mM (252mg/dl) (or lower than 5.5mM (213mg/dl) if arterial disease is already present) by the use of dietary and drug therapy (see *Chapter 9*). Other procedures, such as partial ileal bypass, or LDL-apheresis, can be helpful in the more severe cases (see *Chapter 9*). Regular follow-up is essential to ensure that the level of cholesterol in the blood is maintained within normal limits, and to monitor the onset and progress of any signs of arterial disease.

PLASMA FEATURES OF TYPE IIa HYPERLIPIDAEMIA			
Lipoprotein phenotype	Plasma cholesterol	Plasma triglyceride	Plasma appearance
Type IIa LDL ↑↑↑	elevated	normal	clear, may have increased yellow tint

Fig. 2.38 Characteristic plasma features of Familial Hypercholesterolaemia, Fredrickson Type IIa.

CASE REPORT

A man, aged 35 (Fig. 2.39), presented with arcus juvenalis (Fig. 2.40), and tendon xanthomata over the hands (Fig. 2.41) and elbows (Fig. 2.42). No features of arterial disease were present. However, his family tree showed three first-degree relatives who died of early myocardial infarction, and other members with hypercholesterolaemia (Fig. 2.43). His level of plasma cholesterol at diagnosis was 11.5mM (445mg/dl), but his triglyceride level was normal at 1.5mM

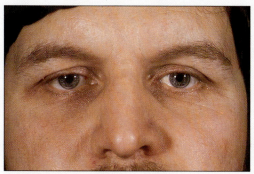

Fig. 2.39 A man, aged 35, with Familial Hypercholesterolaemia, Fredrickson Type IIa.

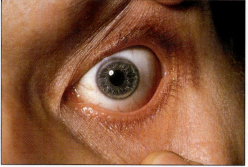

Fig. 2.40 A close-up view of the eye of the patient, showing an arcus juvenalis.

Inherited Defects of Lipid Metabolism

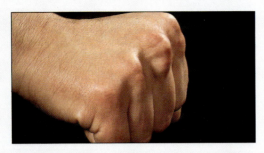

Fig. 2.41 Tendon xanthomata over the hands of the patient.

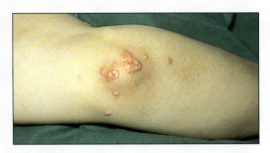

Fig. 2.42 Tendon xanthomata over the elbows of the patient.

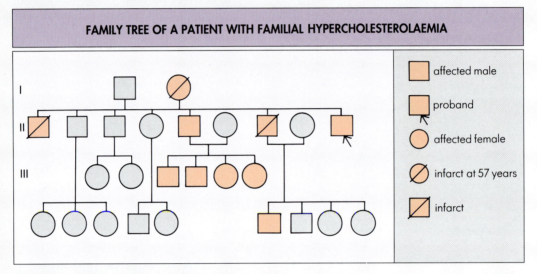

Fig. 2.43 Pedigree of the patient. Note the appearance of an autosomal dominant disease with nearly 50% of members of each generation affected.

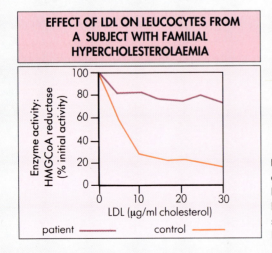

(133mg/dl). Assays of his circulating blood monocytes showed that his LDL receptors could not effectively suppress the activity of the intracellular enzyme, HMGCoA reductase, which is the basic defect in this condition (Fig. 2.44). He died five years later of a myocardial infarct, despite intensive dietary treatment and drug therapy using resins and fibrates.

Fig. 2.44 The effect of LDL on leucocytes, showing a failure to suppress the intracellular enzyme, HMGCoA reductase, in the patient with Familial Hypercholesterolaemia. The control shows normal suppression. Data modified from Higgins M, Galton DJ. *Europ J Clin Invest* 1977;**7**:301.

Disorders of Lipid Transport: The Hyperlipidaemias

Summary of the defects of the lipoprotein cascade

A simple way to summarize the defects in lipoprotein breakdown is illustrated in Fig. 2.45. The transformation of VLDL into LDL with subsequent receptor-mediated clearance by peripheral cells,

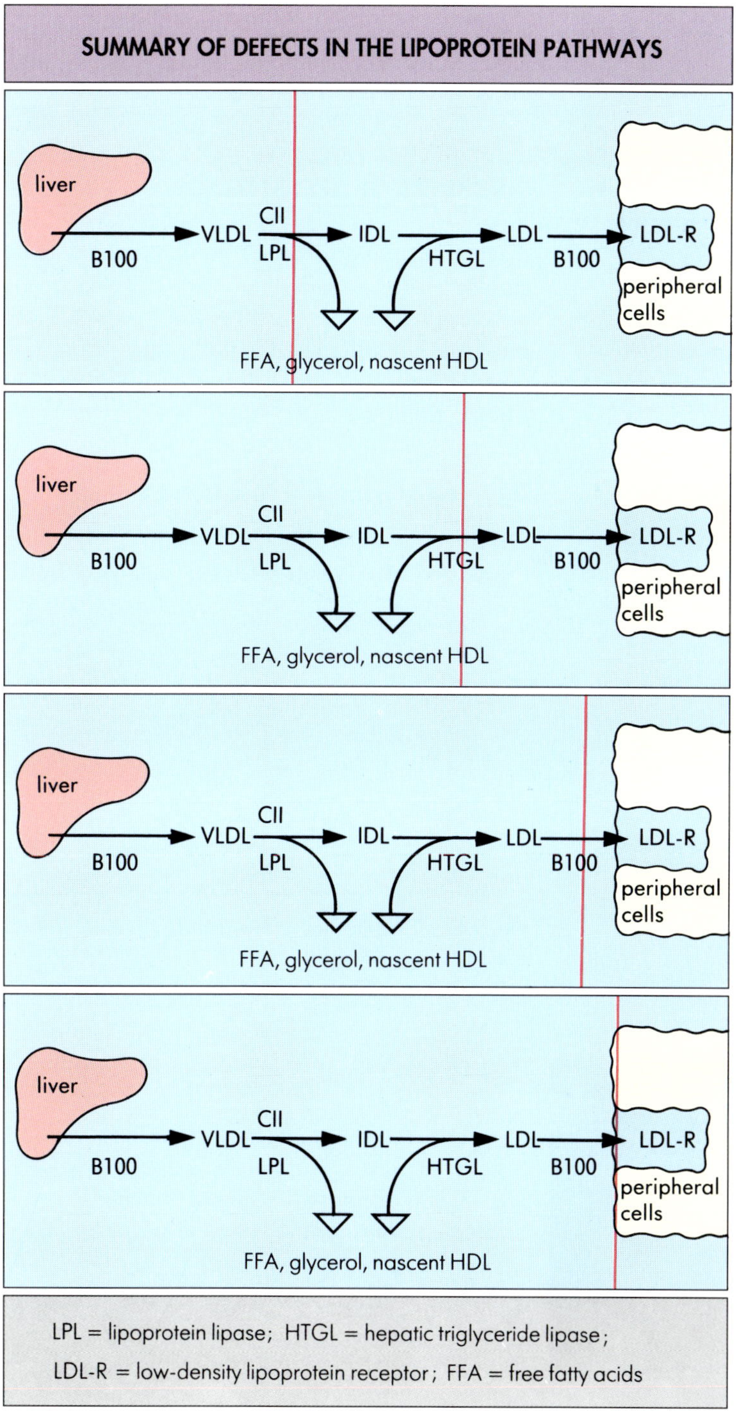

Fig. 2.45 A scheme showing sites of possible defects in the lipoprotein catabolic pathways to produce hypertriglyceridaemia and the combined lipidaemias (see text for full explanation).

LPL = lipoprotein lipase; HTGL = hepatic triglyceride lipase; LDL-R = low-density lipoprotein receptor; FFA = free fatty acids

Inherited Defects of Lipid Metabolism

results in a range of defects which include:
- Defects of either lipoprotein lipase or apolipoprotein CII, which give rise to hypertriglyceridaemia.
- Defects of circulating hepatic lipase which cause accumulation of IDL, resulting in, for example, broad-beta disease.
- Defects at the receptor-binding domain of the B-apolipoprotein, such as the B-100 mutation which leads to accumulation of LDL and a disease resembling Familial Hypercholesterolaemia.
- Defects of the LDL receptor which give rise to Familial Hypercholesterolaemia.

These defects can arise either on a genetic or acquired basis, hence the same lipoprotein phenotype can be produced by a variety of aetiological routes.

Other disorders of apolipoproteins

With the existence of more than eight apolipoproteins, there is a possibility of disorders arising from point mutations or deletions of the relevant genes. Some of these disorders are listed in Fig. 2.46 but will not be discussed further due to their rarity.

DISORDERS OF LIPID STORAGE

Apart from the disorders of lipid transport, there are also a large number of disorders of lipid storage, of which atherosclerosis is the most common and most serious with regard to the health of European populations (Fig. 2.47). Other disorders of lipid storage are rare.

Disorders of lysosomal lipid storage

Of the lysosomal storage disorders, Gaucher's disease is relatively common, particularly in Israel.

SOME RARE APOLIPOPROTEIN DISORDERS	
AI	Tangier disease Milano variant Marburg, Giessen variants Münster 1–3 variants
AIV	Giessen variants Münster variants
B	recessive abetalipoproteinaemia homozygous hypobetalipoproteinaemia B-3500 mutation

Fig. 2.46 Disorders of apolipoproteins which may produce hyperlipidaemia.

DISORDERS OF LIPID STORAGE	
Lysosomal	Nonlysosomal
Gaucher disease Niemann–Pick disease Fabry disease Tay–Sachs (sphingolipidosis)	triglyceride storage disease sitosterol storage atherosclerosis

Fig. 2.47 Classification of the disorders of lipid storage.

CASE REPORT

A patient who had no Jewish antecedents and no family history of Gaucher's disease (Fig. 2.48) was diagnosed as having Gaucher's disease at the age of 27. She had splenomegaly,

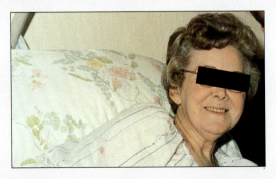

Fig. 2.48 A woman with Gaucher's disease.

Disorders of Lipid Storage

and histology of the spleen showed typical infiltration with Gaucher cells (macrophages which fill up with lysosomal fat to form foam cells) (Fig. 2.49). These foam cells are filled with a complex glycolipid (a glucosylceramide) and gradually invade, replace, and destroy normal tissues. The cells replaced the ends of her humerus, femur, and pelvis, and she developed pathological fractures (Fig. 2.50). She died at the age of 71 after a long, crippling illness.

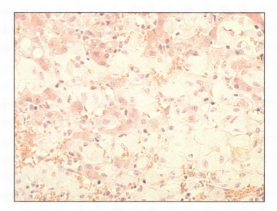

Fig. 2.49 Typical appearances of Gaucher cells (foam-filled macrophages) from the liver of the patient.

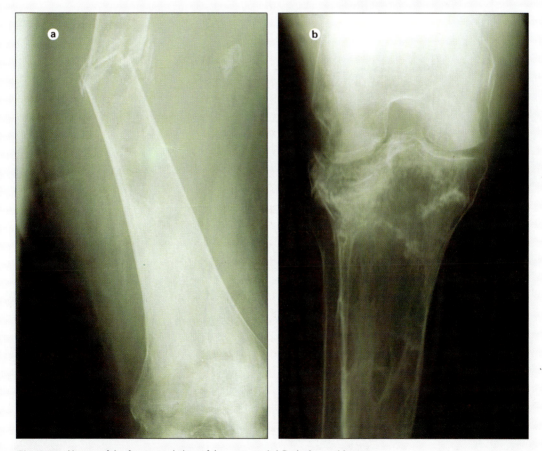

Fig. 2.50 X-rays of the femur and tibia of the patient. (a) Pathological fracture of the femur due to bony replacement with Gaucher cells. (b) Replacement of the head of the tibia with Gaucher cells.

Inherited Defects of Lipid Metabolism

Disorders of nonlysosomal lipid storage

The nonlysosomal storage disorders are of more relevance to atherosclerosis. Abnormal storage of triglyceride can occur in the tissues around the neck (Fig. 2.51) and in the peripheral subcutaneous tissues of the hands, despite the gross emaciation of the rest of the body (Fig. 2.52). This latter storage defect gives rise to a bimodal distribution of adipose-cell diameters between the hands and abdomen (Fig. 2.53). Defects in the breakdown of intracellular triglyceride in the abnormal tissue occurs in both cases (Fig. 2.54). Although such nonlysosomal storage disorders are rare, their pathophysiology may help to elucidate some aspects of the abnormal storage of lipid in the arterial wall which produces atherosclerosis. Study of such rare defects can help to identify rate-determining steps in the pathological process, which may also be altered in the commoner forms of disease.

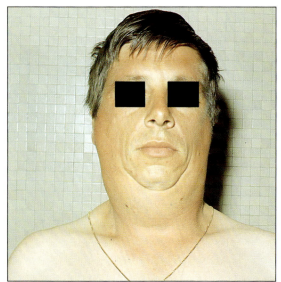 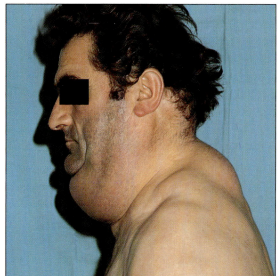

Fig. 2.51 Two patients with abnormal storage of fat in the tissues around the neck.

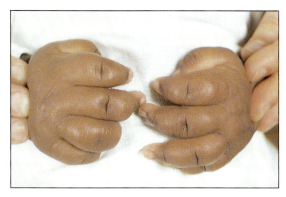 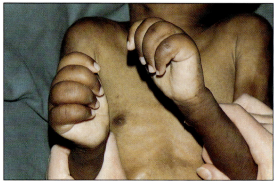

Fig. 2.52 (a) Abnormal storage of triglycerides in the peripheral subcutaneous tissues of the hand of an infant. (b) Close-up view of the hands showing abnormal storage of lipids.

Disorders of Lipid Storage

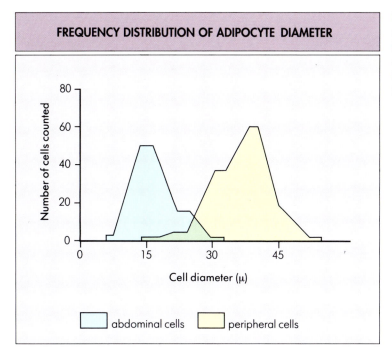

Fig. 2.53 Bimodal distribution of adipose-cell diameters between the hands and abdomen of the patient in *Fig. 2.52*. Data modified from Galton DJ, Reckless JPD, Taitz J. *Act Paed Scand* 1976;**65**:761.

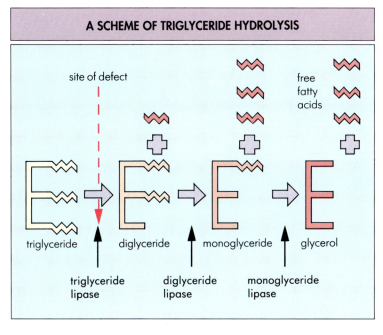

Fig. 2.54 A scheme of triglyceride hydrolysis and site of defects in patients with triglyceride-storage disorders.

45

CHAPTER THREE

The New Genetics

There has been a recent revolution in the study of genetics of the common inherited disorders of metabolism. The study of clinical genetics previously involved discovering a mutant protein, and subsequently carrying out studies on the co-segregation of the protein with the disease in pedigrees. This has now changed since the discovery of the great amount of genetic variation that occurs within, and adjacent to genes that can be identified by restriction endonucleases (enzymes that can cut the DNA helix at specific points). When used in the method of Southern blotting, endonucleases reveal restriction fragment-length polymorphisms (RFLP's) of genomic DNA which can be used as

Fig. 3.1 Clinical genetics: New developments.

CLINICAL GENETICS: NEW DEVELOPMENTS		
	Old	New
Study	rare mutant subjects	any organism
Basic tools	mutant proteins	restriction fragment-length polymorphisms
Map by	recombination in pedigrees	ordered cDNA library
Function by	complementation	deduction from protein structure
Treatment	replace or restrict gene product	replace gene (if possible)

markers for any gene in the vicinity. The advances of the new genetics enable analysis of almost any inherited condition to be carried out (Fig. 3.1). Attempts can also be made to determine the location of the gene, and to deduce the function of the gene product from the DNA and RNA structure. This can be of great use in the study of lipaemias and atherosclerosis (Fig. 3.2). The presence of susceptibility genes are not sufficient to cause the development of these diseases; however, interaction with environmental factors, such as high animal-fat diets or obesity, can cause the diseases to become manifest. The new genetics enables determination of the location of these susceptibility genes (represented by the inner circles of the Venn diagram in Fig. 3.2), thus allowing early identification of individuals who are at risk, and will also stimulate the search for new therapeutic agents that may block or interfere with the action of such predisposition genes.

CANDIDATE GENES

Over 1.4 million potential genes exist in the human genome (Fig. 3.3). However, which of these genes may be involved in the inheritance of the common hyperlipidaemias and premature atherosclerosis, still remains to be determined. The extent to which premature atherosclerosis is inherited can be calculated from studies of identical twins by observing how many twin pairs both develop early arterial disease; this turns out to be approximately 65% (that is, of the monozygotic twin pairs studied, 65% are concordant for the disease). The genes which code for the apolipoproteins and lipoprotein receptors, and which have been found to be abnormally expressed in both quality and quantity in atherosclerosis, are the first candidates to consider in the search for the major genes involved in

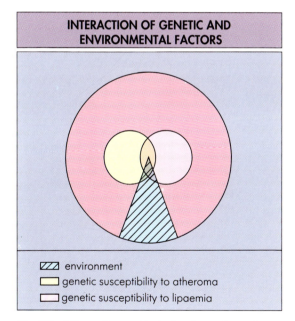

Fig. 3.2 A Venn diagram illustrating the pathogenic factors for atherosclerosis. The outer circle represents a population containing subgroups (inner circles) of individuals genetically predisposed to atheroma or hyperlipidaemia. The hatched sector represents individuals exposed to a particular environmental factor such as high dietary intake of cholesterol.

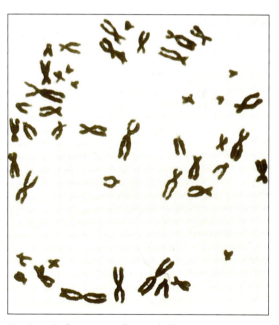

Fig. 3.3 A chromosomal spread. The 44 autosomes and the two sex chromosomes are shown.

the inheritance of premature atherosclerosis (Fig. 3.4). Other relevant genes may include those coding for arterial-wall proteins, and those coding for hormonal and/or other growth factors.

A great amount of progress has been made in identifying all the lipid-related genes in the human chromosomes, and in determining their map locations (Fig. 3.5). These genes are dispersed amongst seven chromosomes, although not quite at random.

CANDIDATE GENES FOR ATHEROSCLEROSIS				
Lipids	Clotting factors	Hormones	Arterial-wall components	Other diseases
cholesterol LDL HDL Lp (a)	fibrinogen plasminogen factor VII platelets	insulin growth factors oestrogens	cells endothelial macrophages smooth-muscle	diabetes hypertension
triglyceride VLDL IDL			protein matrix fibronectin glycosamino- glycans collagen	obesity smoking stress response
receptors LDL remnant HDL				
apolipoproteins A,B,C,E				

Fig. 3.4 Candidate genes for atherosclerosis. These phenotypic factors have been considered as abnormal in the early development of the atherosclerotic plaque. The new genetics can help to determine which of these factors are inherited, and which are secondary to the development of atheroma.

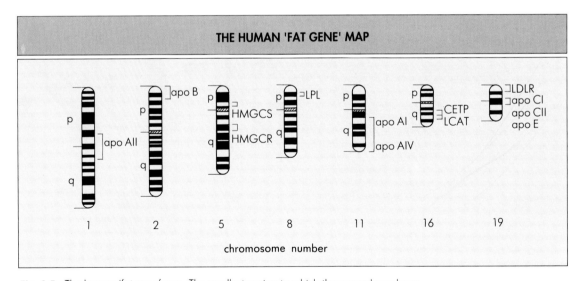

Fig. 3.5 The human 'fat gene' map. The smallest region to which the genes have been assigned is indicated by brackets. Apo = apolipoprotein; HMGCS = hydroxymethylglutaryl CoA synthase; HMGCR = hydroxymethylglutaryl CoA reductase; LPL = lipoprotein lipase; CETP = cholesterol ester transfer protein; LCAT = lecithin:cholesterol acyltransferase; LDLR = LDL receptor. Modified from Lusis J, Sparkes RS. *Monographs Human Genetics* 1989;**12**:79.

GENE CLUSTERS

Closer inspection of the chromosomes reveals that there are two main clusters of the apolipoprotein genes: one cluster is present on chromosome 11 and the other, on chromosome 19 (Fig. 3.6). This suggests that these clusters may have evolved from a single ancestral gene by duplication and subsequent dispersion amongst the different chromosomes. The structures of all the apolipoprotein genes have been elucidated and compared in order to examine this possibility. A prototype gene (Fig. 3.7) consists of a 5' regulatory sequence, often containing a TATA box, a start codon which initiates mRNA synthesis, and a number of intervening sequences or introns which divide the coding region of the gene into exons; the end of the gene often has a polyadenine tail. By comparing the various structures of the apolipoprotein genes, it can be seen that they all possess three introns in

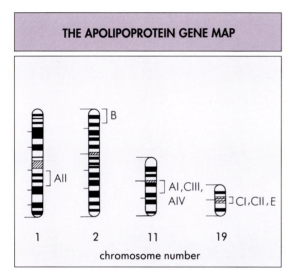

Fig. 3.6 Chromosomal localization of the apolipoprotein multigene family. This map of human chromosomes 1, 2, 11, and 19, shows approximate assignments of the apolipoprotein genes. The apolipoproteins AI, AII, CI, and so on, are at the corresponding gene loci.

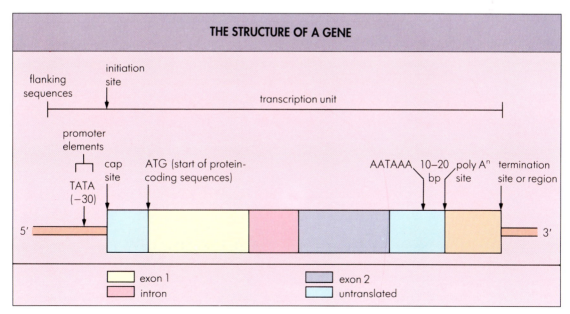

Fig. 3.7 A prototype gene showing the basic elements.

similar positions: one in the 5′ untranslated region, one in the leader sequence, and one in the coding sequence (Fig. 3.8). The genes are thus divided into four exons. The genes may have 'evolved' from the smallest of the apolipoprotein genes, apolipoprotein CI, by gene duplication and expansion of 22 codons in exons 3 or 4 (Fig. 3.9). It is likely that during evolution, the apolipoprotein genes have dispersed from chromosome 19 to others, since another gene cluster is found on chromosome 11, and another gene (the gene for apolipoprotein AII), is found on its own on chromosome 1. The intron–exon structure of the gene for apolipoprotein B on the tip of chromosome 2 suggests that it does not form part of this multigene family.

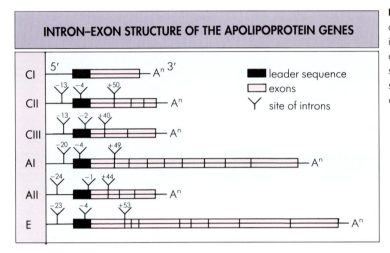

Fig. 3.8 Genomic structures of the apolipoprotein multigene family. The intron–exon organization of members of the apolipoprotein gene family is shown. The numbers above the intron sites are base pairs from the start codon.

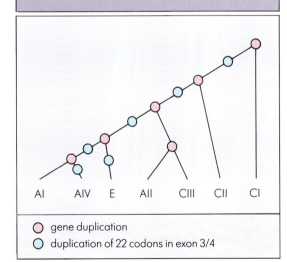

Fig. 3.9 A hypothetical scheme for the evolution of the apolipoprotein genes. The ancestral gene was probably similar to apolipoprotein CI. Gene duplication led to the evolution of apolipoprotein CII. Duplication of 22 codons in exon 3 or 4 diversified the length.

GENETIC DIVERSITY

The apolipoprotein genes show a great deal of nucleotide diversity; for example, in the apolipoprotein AI–CIII–AIV gene cluster on chromosome 11, there are more than eight sites which produce polymorphic variants when digested with restriction endonucleases (Fig. 3.10), and it has been calculated that approximately 1 in every 500 nucleotide bases in flanking regions may be variable. In the gene cluster on chromosome 19, some of this genetic variation in the coding region of the gene for apolipoprotein E produces polymorphic proteins, that is, the variation affects the coding sequence of the E gene to yield different peptides. The main sites of this variation involve amino acids at positions 112 and 158, producing E variants termed E4 and E2, respectively (if E3 is considered as the ancestral protein) (Figs 3.11 and 3.12). Different E-apolipoproteins are associated with different levels of cholesterol in world populations, so this genetic variation may be functionally important.

Gene Diversity

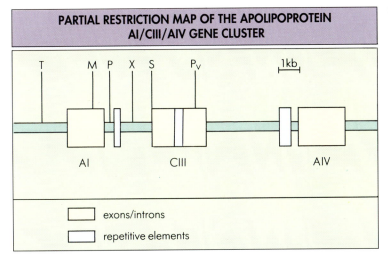

PARTIAL RESTRICTION MAP OF THE APOLIPOPROTEIN AI/CIII/AIV GENE CLUSTER

Fig. 3.10 Restriction map of the AI/CIII/AIV genes showing multiple polymorphic sites. Pv,Pvu,PvuII; Sst 1; X, Xmn1; P, Pst 1; M, Msp 1; T, Taq 1, are sites that digest with the appropriate restriction enzymes.

GENETIC POLYMORPHISMS OF APOLIPOPROTEIN E

E4 — arginine
         ↑ 112   158
E3 — cysteine   arginine
                  145   ↓
E2 — arginine   cysteine
         ↓
E2* — cysteine

Fig. 3.11 Amino-acid substitutions in the commonly occurring genetic polymorphisms of apolipoprotein E, producing more than three different proteins (E2, E3, E4, E2*)

HUMAN APOLIPOPROTEIN-E POLYMORPHISMS

Name	Charge difference	Defect
E7	+4	unknown
E5	+2	unknown
E4	+1	$Cys_{112} \to Arg$
E3	0	—
E3*	0	$Ala_{99} \to Thr$, $Ala_{152} \to Pro$
E3**	0	$Cys_{112} \to Arg$, $Arg_{142} \to Cys$
E2	−1	$Arg_{158} \to Cys$
E2*	−1	$Arg_{145} \to Cys$
E2**	−1	$Lys_{146} \to Gln$
E1	−2	$Gly_{127} \to Asp$, $Arg_{158} \to Cys$

Fig. 3.12 Polymorphism of the human apolipoprotein-E protein showing many other different variants that have been identified.

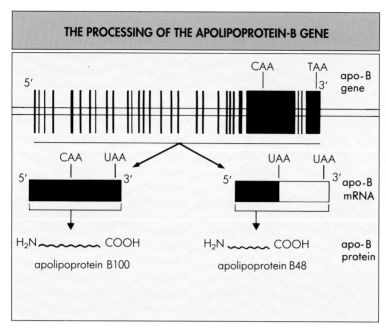

Fig. 3.13 A diagram of the gene for apolipoprotein B, and the processing of intestinal and liver mRNA and B-apolipoproteins. Two separate mRNAs are synthesized from the gene for apolipoprotein B, one containing the CAA codon for glutamine, present in apolipoprotein B100, and the other containing the premature stop codon which codes for apolipoprotein B48. Modified from Scott J, Wallis SC et al. In: Suckling KE, Groot PH, eds. *Hyperlipidaemia of Atherosclerosis.* London: Academic Press, 1988:47.

A particularly interesting genetic variation has been observed in the apolipoprotein-B gene (Fig. 3.13). The gene for apolipoprotein B makes two different proteins, a B-100 product and a B-48 product which is approximately half the size of the former. Two peptides are usually made from a single gene by alternatively 'splicing out' some of the internal exons. In the case of apolipoprotein B48, the mRNA of B100 is edited to transform a CAA codon for glutamine (present in B100) into UAA (a stop codon). The synthesis of the protein terminates at this stage, and the smaller peptide, apolipoprotein B48, is produced. This smaller apolipoprotein does not carry the LDL-receptor binding domain, and its function remains to be determined.

EVOLUTION AND GENETIC VARIATION

The distribution of the previously described genetic variants amongst the world populations depends on many different evolutionary forces (Fig. 3.14). Perhaps the two most important forces are directional selection (either in favour of spread of the gene variant or its extinction), and genetic drift. Directional selection depends on the functional effects of the genetic variation, the process of natural selection tending to eliminate variants which have an adverse effect on survival, or it favours the spread of the variants which have a beneficial effect. The process of genetic drift is a different phenomenon which influences gene frequencies. The gene frequency can change due to random selection of genetic variants from one generation to the next. A special example of this is the increase in frequency of a rare genetic variant in a localized population, due to the 'founder' effect. This can be due to migration of a 'founder' genotype into a sparsely populated locality, and its spread by differential reproduction. A good example of the 'founder' effect is the gene for the rare metabolic disease, Variegate Porphyria, which was probably introduced into South Africa by a Dutch immigrant in 1688, and subsequently spread in the white and black populations, affecting approximately 1 in every 330 births. This disease was probably spread by the 'founder' effect, despite the undoubted selective disadvantage which is associated with this genotype.

Balanced polymorphism is another principal mechanism which maintains two genetic variants in a population; the homozygous genotype may confer a selective disadvantage, while the hetero-

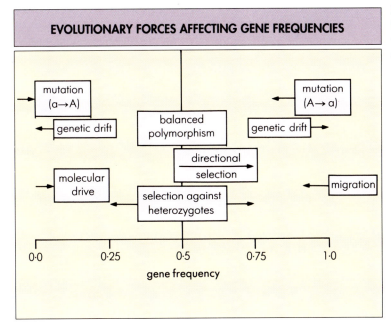

Fig. 3.14 The major evolutionary forces which affect gene frequencies, the two most important being directional selection and genetic drift.

zygous state confers a selective advantage. A good example of balanced polymorphism is sickle-cell anaemia (the homozygous state) which is maintained in the populations of West Africa by the selective survival value of sickle-cell trait (the heterozygous state) affording protection against malaria.

GENETIC MARKERS

Genetic variations can be used to localize possible gene defects for the common metabolic disorders such as hyperlipidaemia or atherosclerosis, by two essential strategies: population genetics and pedigree genetics (Fig. 3.15). Generally speaking, the two approaches are complementary. Population genetics is a good approach for screening loci to see if they might be involved in the inherited predisposition to the disease. If this approach provides positive results, then the approach of pedigree genetics can be pursued in order to attempt to define further, and eventually sequence, the aetiological mutation. This involves much more work than the population strategy in that complete pedigrees have to be assembled for cosegregation analysis of affected members, using

STRATEGIES TO DEFINE GENETIC DEFECTS

Population genetics	Pedigree genetics
disease-association studies	linkage analysis
easy-to-ascertain subjects	difficult to assemble all family members
control group is critical	controls within the pedigree
candiate-gene approach	candidate gene or random polymorphic marker
information for ~ 100kb around linkage marker (0.1–0.5% recombination fraction)	information for ~ 15,000kb around marker

Fig. 3.15 Strategies to define genetic defects.

possible DNA markers. The aim of the population strategy is illustrated in Fig. 3.16. It is known that rare mutants of lipoprotein lipase or apolipoprotein CII can produce hypertriglyceridaemia, but these mutants account for very little of the common hypertriglyceridaemias seen in a lipid clinic. There are likely to be more common polymorphic genes that predispose to the development of lipaemia, and these can be located by the use of genetic variations in their vicinity. At present, two types of genetic variations are commonly used (Fig. 3.17).

In one type of DNA polymorphism, a single nucleotide, adjacent to the candidate gene, is variable so that the restriction endonuclease no longer cuts at this site but uses the next one along. This restriction-site polymorphism (point mutation) involves nucleotide substitutions, and yields two distinct alleles which are 2kb and 3kb in size in Fig. 3.17; these alleles can be used to determine whether there is an unequal distribution of them between patient and matched-control groups. If this is the case, this would suggest that a nearby gene contributes to the inheritance of the disorder.

An alternative and very useful DNA polymorphism involves a hypervariable DNA sequence which causes a variable amount of DNA to be inserted at the polymorphic locus. On digestion with restriction enzymes, fragments of variable size are produced depending on the amount of DNA inserted at the site. This often allows positive identification of the parental genes, and enables their tracking in pedigrees and populations.

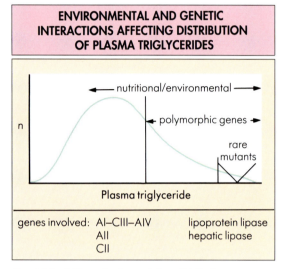

Fig. 3.16 A theoretical population distribution curve for a blood nutrient. This illustrates the role of rare mutant genes and common polymorphic gene variants interacting with environmental factors, which account for the right-hand side of the distribution curve.

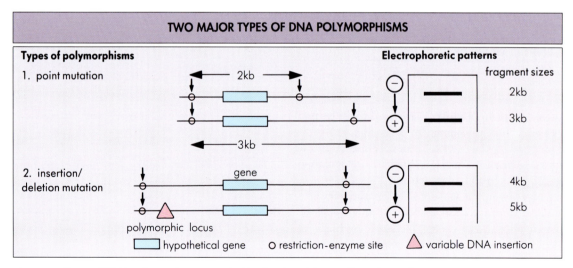

Fig. 3.17 Types of DNA polymorphisms revealed by Southern blotting. This scheme illustrates a hypothetical gene digested with the restriction enzyme, together with the blotting patterns after gel electrophoresis of the DNA fragments. One type of polymorphism is due to nucleotide substitutions (panel 1). The other is due to variable DNA insertions at the polymorphic locus (panel 2).

Genetic Markers

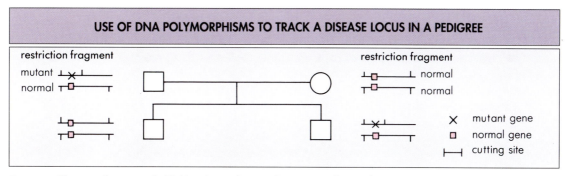

Fig. 3.18 The use of nonspecific DNA polymorphisms adjacent to a disease locus to track its transmission through a pedigree. A restriction-site polymorphism is used to track a mutant gene in a pedigree. There are two cutting sites for the restriction enzyme, close to the mutant gene, but only one is close to the normal gene. The difference in the size of the fragments can be easily detected on Southern blotting, and allows identification of offspring to whom the mutant gene has been transmitted.

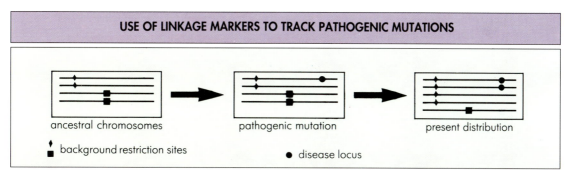

Fig. 3.19 The use of linkage markers to identify possible aetiological gene loci.

Pedigree genetics

Restriction fragment-length polymorphisms are used in pedigree genetics to see if mutant genes track with affected members (Fig. 3.18). It should be remembered that these restriction fragment-length polymorphisms are only linkage markers (Fig. 3.19): they may be background ancestral mutations that mainly have no functional significance, but are close to an aetiological mutation for which they can act as markers. However, the marker sites can cross over with other ones during meiosis so that the pathogenic mutation may not be exclusively flagged by the adjacent polymorphic site. The closer the marker site is to the aetiological mutation, the less chance there is for crossover to occur, and the more general its use as a marker in studies of population or pedigree genetics.

A more complex three-generation pedigree is illustrated in Fig. 3.20, where two alleles, L and S,

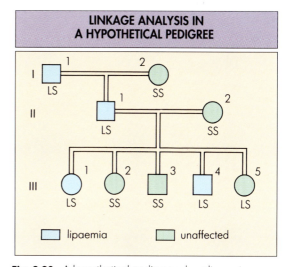

Fig. 3.20 A hypothetical pedigree where lipaemic members are segregating, and individuals are genotyped for markers (L and S alleles). All affected members possess an L allele, except III5 (See text for explanation).

are identified by restriction-enzyme analysis. The L allele tracks with diseased members except for member III5 who possesses the L allele (but is unaffected). This may either be due to a crossover event during meiosis, causing the L marker to dissociate from the aetiological mutation, or alternatively, the hypothesis (that the L allele marks the disease) may be incorrect. There are complex statistical techniques (such as the LOD score), which help to decide between these issues. An example in practice is illustrated by the pedigree in Fig. 3.21 where hypercholesterolaemia is segregating in some family members. The allele labelled disease V1 in Fig. 3.21 can be identified from the Southern blot technique (Fig. 3.22) showing that the 19-kb fragment (the V1 allele) is distinct from the 16-kb fragment (the V2 allele). When these alleles are traced through the pedigree of *Fig. 3.21*, it can be seen that a V1 allele tracks with affected members exclusively and provides presumptive evidence that the adjacent gene, the LDL receptor in this case, is the aetiological locus.

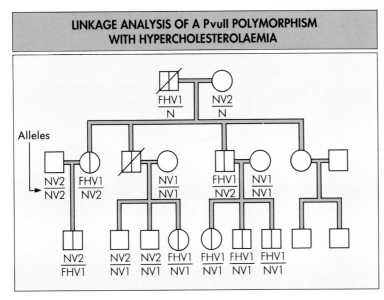

Fig. 3.21 A pedigree in which hypercholesterolaemia is segregating. Members have been genotyped using a PvuII polymorphism, and it is seen that all affected members possess a V1 allele. Data modified from Humphries SE, Kessling AM, Horsthemke B, Seed M, Jowett NI, Holm M, Galton DJ *et al. Lancet* 1985;**i**:1003. FHV1 = allele associated with hypercholesterolaemia; NV1 = allele not associated with hypercholesterolaemia.

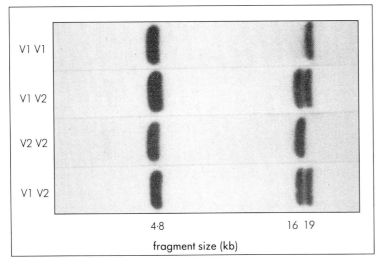

Fig. 3.22 Southern blot of the PvuII polymorphism of the LDL-receptor gene which is used to genotype the members of the pedigree in *Fig. 3.21*.

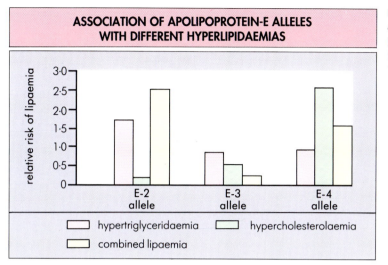

Fig. 3.23 The association of different apolipoprotein-E alleles with the hyperlipidaemias. Modified from Utermann G. *CIBA Symposium* 1987;**130**:52.

Population genetics

DNA markers can be used to study the hyperlipidaemias in populations, a good example of this being the study of the polymorphisms of the E-apolipoprotein. In Caucasian populations, there is a 2.5-fold increase in hypercholesterolaemia in individuals possessing the E4 protein when compared to subjects with the E2 protein (who have a lower level of blood cholesterol than that of the mean population). Conversely, subjects with the E2 protein have an almost two-fold increase in hypertriglyceridaemia when compared to subjects with the E3 protein (Fig. 3.23). Other genetic variants at different loci, such as the apolipoprotein AI–CIII–AIV gene cluster on chromosome 11, are also known to influence the levels of plasma lipids.

METHODS USED TO STUDY GENETIC VARIATION

The Southern blotting procedure

The technique of Southern blotting has been widely used in order to detect genetic variations at candidate loci, although newer methods are currently being developed to replace this cumbersome procedure. In this technique, genomic DNA is isolated from leucocytes in a 10–15ml sample of blood: the DNA is digested with restriction enzymes, and the fragments are run out on agarose gel using electrophoresis (Fig. 3.24). The fragments are then transferred from the gel to nitrocellulose filters where they are hybridized with P^{32}-labelled gene probes. The latter hybridize with their complementary strands of DNA and locate them after subjection to autoradiography. The technique allows identification of the number of genes present in the genome (that is, the copy number), as well as the size of the restriction fragment on which the gene is carried (by determining the distance the fragment has moved into the gel). When mutations occur at the sites of action of restriction endonucleases, the fragment size varies, and this provides the basis of linkage markers.

The polymerase chain reaction

The polymerase chain reaction is a technique which amplifies stretches of DNA for detailed analysis such as DNA sequencing (Fig. 3.25). Two primers are bound at the end of the stretch of DNA of interest, and a copy of this DNA is built up from the primer. After the copy has been made, the fragments are separated, new primer is added, and the cycle of building up further copies from the primer recommences. In this way, there is an exponential increase in the amount of the DNA sequence located between the primers.

The New Genetics

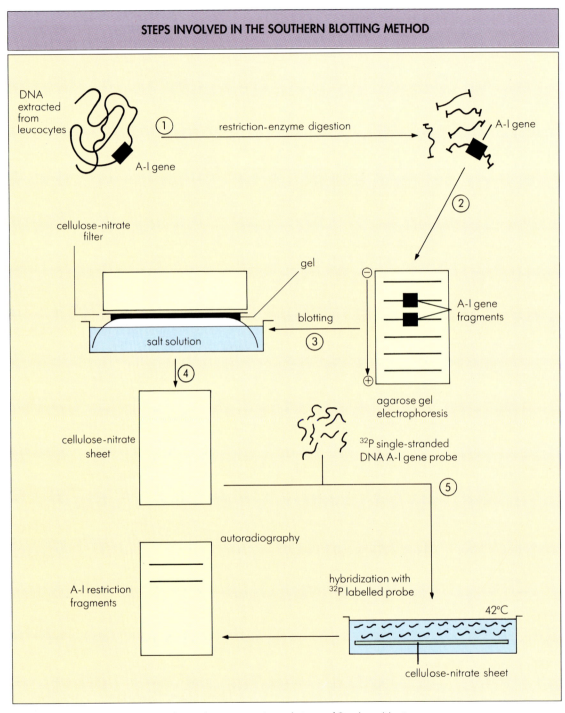

Fig. 3.24 Detection of genetic polymorphisms using the technique of Southern blotting. The basic steps involve digestion of patient's DNA with restriction enzymes; gel electrophoresis of DNA fragments; and hybridization with a ^{32}P-labelled gene probe.

Methods Used to Study Genetic Variation

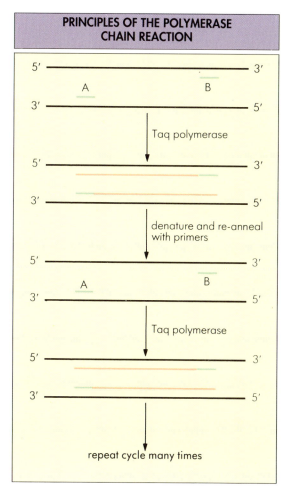

Fig. 3.25 Gene amplification by the polymerase chain reaction. Primers (A and B) are used to make copies of the DNA sequence of interest and the cycle is repeated many times to build up large amounts of DNA.

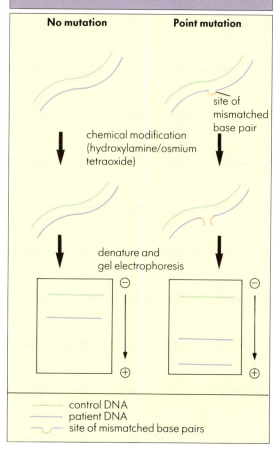

Fig. 3.26 Base-pair mismatch and cleavage. The patient's DNA is hybridized to control DNA, and sites of mismatch of base pairs make the DNA strand susceptible to cleavage by chemical agents. This may identify aetiological mutations in the patient's genes.

Base-pair mismatches

Identification of critical mutations in a stretch of DNA from patients is often necessary. This can be achieved by hybridizing the DNA from the patient with control DNA in order to determine if any base-pair differences exist (Fig. 3.26). Mismatched base pairs are susceptible to chemical cleavage by agents, such as hydroxylamine and osmium tetraoxide. The fragments produced by cleavage can then be run out on gels, and the position of the base-pair mismatches can be identified by the size of the fragments. The position of the base-pair mismatch may be the site of the aetiological mutation. This technique is very useful in providing a fine structural analysis of mutations in exon or regulatory sequences, without having to undertake an extensive programme of DNA sequencing.

CHAPTER FOUR

Epidemiology of Blood Lipids and Atherosclerosis

The number of deaths which occur in Northern Europe due to coronary heart disease is greater than the total number due to all the cancers (Fig. 4.1). The difference is even greater if cases of

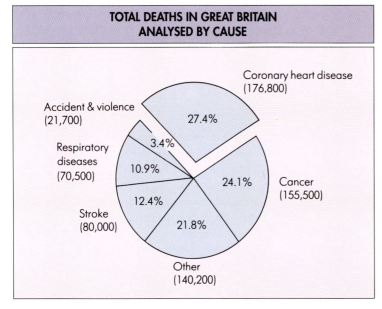

Fig. 4.1 Total deaths in Great Britain. Source: Annual abstracts of statistics 1986, data.

stroke are included in the group with coronary heart disease, since a proportion of strokes arise on the basis of cerebrovascular atherosclerosis. There is a widespread variation in mortality rates in men due to coronary heart disease amongst various countries (Fig. 4.2). This variation is generally related to the mean levels of blood cholesterol of the different populations (Fig. 4.3). If the two sets of data are combined, a good linear relationship between mean total blood cholesterol and relative incidence of coronary heart disease amongst world populations can be seen (Fig. 4.4). Individuals from the population of rural China have the lowest mean blood cholesterol of 3.3mM (130mg/dl), and the mean mortality rates due to coronary heart disease in middle-aged individuals are approximately 5% of those in Great Britain.

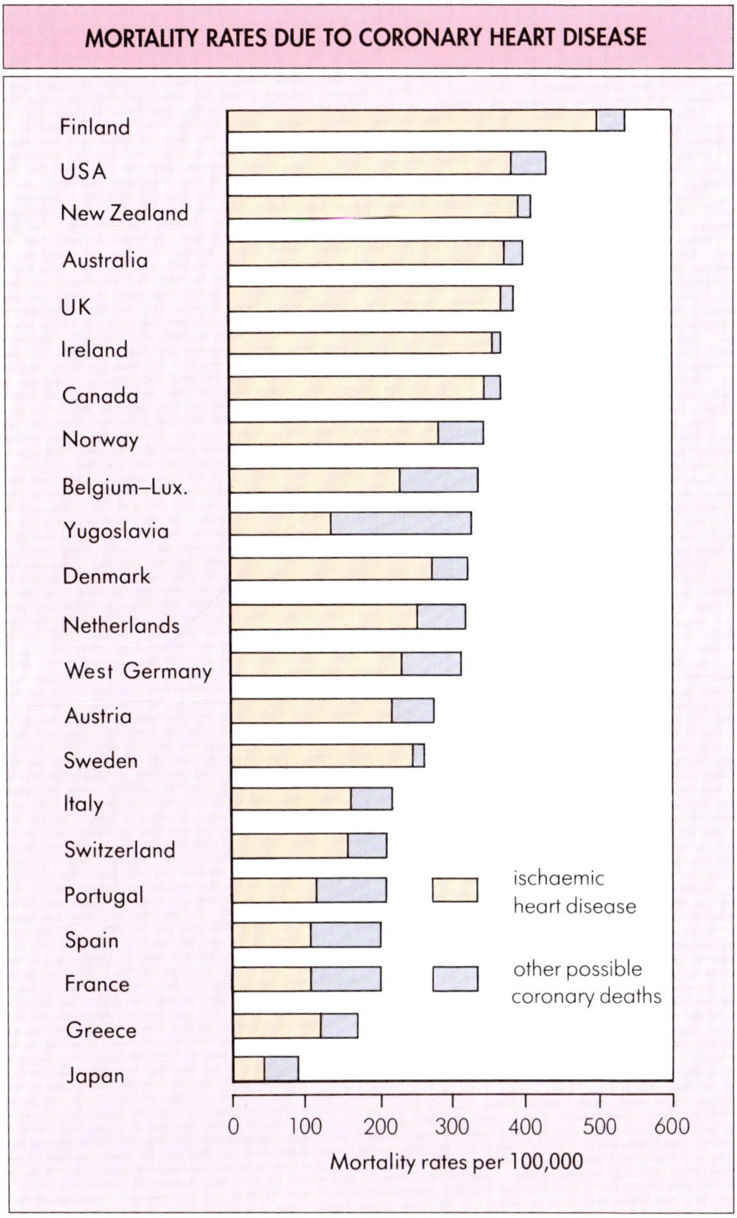

MORTALITY RATES DUE TO CORONARY HEART DISEASE

Finland	
USA	
New Zealand	
Australia	
UK	
Ireland	
Canada	
Norway	
Belgium–Lux.	
Yugoslavia	
Denmark	
Netherlands	
West Germany	
Austria	
Sweden	
Italy	
Switzerland	
Portugal	
Spain	
France	
Greece	
Japan	

Mortality rates per 100,000

- ischaemic heart disease
- other possible coronary deaths

Fig. 4.2 Mortality rates in men aged 35–64 amongst various countries, due to coronary heart disease (age-standardized rates). Data modified from Richard JL. *Atherosclerosis* 1984; **VI**:821.

Epidemiology of Blood Lipids and Atherosclerosis

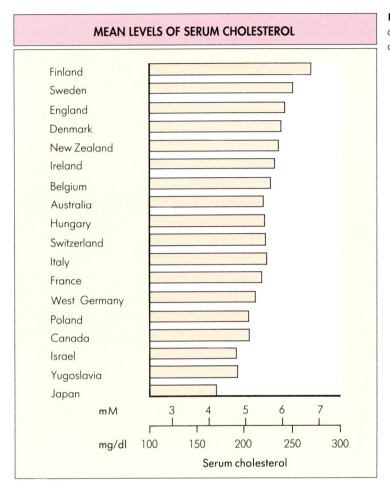

Fig. 4.3 Mean levels of serum cholesterol of men in different countries.

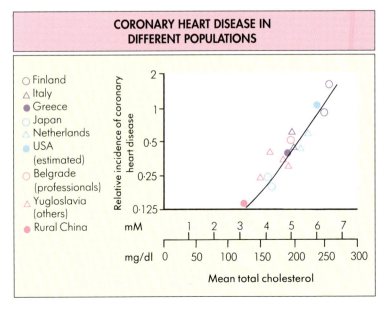

Fig. 4.4 Incidence of coronary heart disease related to levels of mean total cholesterol in different populations. Data modified from Keys A *et al. Ann Int Med* 1958;**48**:83.

POPULATION STUDIES

Many population studies have confirmed the relationship of the level of blood lipids with the incidence of coronary artery disease.

The Framingham Study

The Framingham Study was one of the earliest studies that prospectively followed the citizens of Framingham, Massachusetts, for more than 20 years. The study revealed a significant relationship between the level of serum cholesterol and the risk of coronary heart disease (Fig. 4.5). The ratio of total-cholesterol:HDL-cholesterol (or LDL-cholesterol:HDL-cholesterol) was also found to be significantly related to the risk of coronary heart disease (Fig. 4.6). Furthermore, there was a significant relationship between plasma triglyceride levels and coronary heart disease in subjects

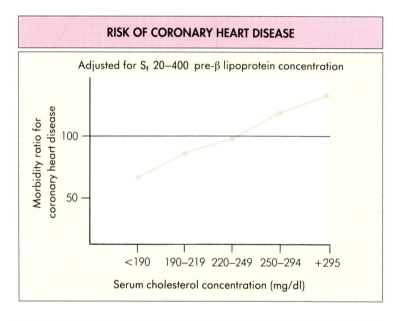

Fig. 4.5 The Framingham Study: Risk of coronary heart disease (14 years) follow-up in men aged 38–69, according to serum lipids adjusted for associated variables. Data modified from Kannel WB, Castelli WP, Gordon T, McNamara PM. *Ann Int Med* 1971;**74**:1.

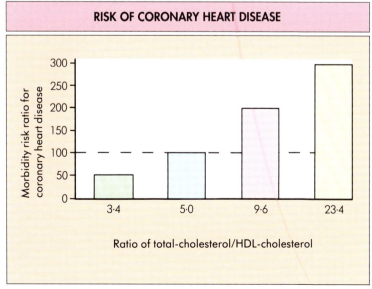

Fig. 4.6 The Framingham Study: Four-year risk of coronary heart disease according to the ratio of cholesterol lipoprotein fractions. Data modified from Kannel WB. *Nutrition Rev* 1988;**46**:68.

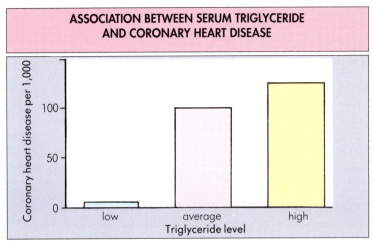

Fig. 4.7 The Framingham Study: The association between the levels of serum triglyceride and incidence of coronary heart disease in men with low levels of HDL-cholesterol <1.0mM (40mg/dl); low triglyceride <1.1mM (94mg/dl); average triglyceride 1.1–1.6mM (94–114mg/dl); high triglyceride >1.6mM (>145mg/dl). Data modified from Castelli WP. *Am Heart J* 1986;**112**:432.

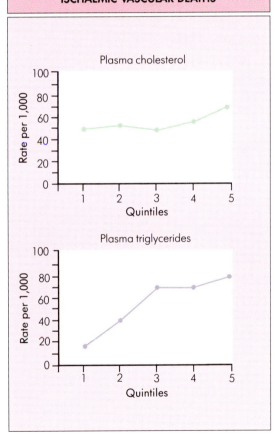

Fig. 4.8 The Stockholm Prospective Study: Rate per 1,000 of ischaemic vascular deaths in the different quintiles of plasma cholesterol and triglyceride distributions. Data modified from Carlson LA, Bottiger LE. *Acta Med Scan* 1985;**218**:207.

with low levels of HDL (Fig. 4.7). Many other epidemiological studies have confirmed and extended these observations. Other studies, such as the Stockholm Prospective Study, have found that high levels of triglyceride-rich lipoproteins are independent risk factors for coronary heart disease. The Framingham Study did not initially support this observation, but more recent data (when combined with HDL levels) pointed to the same conclusion.

The Stockholm Prospective Study

The Stockholm Prospective Study involved the prospective study of 3,486 men, for 14.5 years, who were attending a health centre in Sweden. The end point of the study was proven myocardial infarction or ischaemic vascular death. An interesting finding from this study was that high levels of plasma triglycerides constituted a major independent risk factor for the development of arterial disease (Fig. 4.8), whereas a high level of plasma cholesterol appeared to be a less-strong risk factor. The reasons for this are not clear but may relate to ethnic, environmental, or geographical differences.

The Oslo Heart Study

The Oslo Heart Study was a study of the risk factors involved in coronary heart disease amongst men in Oslo, aged 40–49 years. The coronary and main intracranial arteries of the men who died were collected at autopsy and examined for raised atherosclerotic lesions. The results showed that levels of total serum cholesterol, blood pressure, and levels of fasting serum triglycerides, significantly correlated to raised atherosclerotic lesions; HDL-cholesterol was negatively correlated to such lesions (Fig. 4.9).

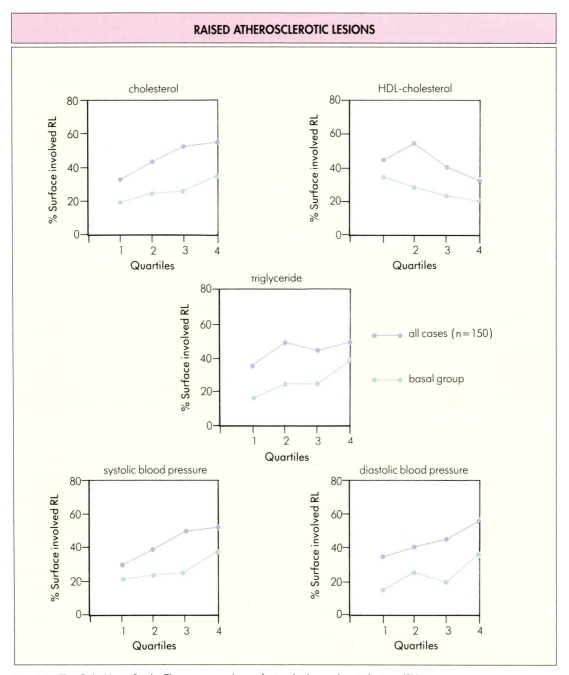

Fig. 4.9 The Oslo Heart Study: The mean numbers of raised atherosclerotic lesions (RL) in all cases (n=150) and in a basal group of cases, by increasing values of risk factors. Data modified from Solberg LA, Enger SC et al. Atherosclerosis 1980;**V**:57.

Epidemiology of Blood Lipids and Atherosclerosis

The Multiple Risk Factor Intervention Trial

The Multiple Risk Factor Intervention Trial (MRFIT) is a study that is often quoted and which involved individuals with several risk factors for coronary heart disease, including elevated levels of cholesterol, smoking, and high blood pressure. More than 300,000 men were recruited to the trial in order to study the effects of various therapeutic factors on future coronary events: these included dietary intervention on levels of blood cholesterol, drug therapy for hypertension, and special advice to dissuade individuals from smoking. Intervention did not appear to be very effective. However, there was a curvilinear relationship between the levels of serum cholesterol and death rates from coronary heart disease (Fig. 4.10), no threshold effect being observed. There was a gradient of risk that increased as the level of cholesterol was elevated. This study has given rise to the widely accepted limits of blood cholesterol levels of 5.2–6.5mM (200–250mg/dl) which require dietary therapy, and those above 6.5mM (250mg/dl) which are likely to require additional drug therapy. It should be pointed out that if these limits were adopted for the UK, approximately 30–40% of the entire population would be 'on treatment', so such strict criteria may not be practicable at present.

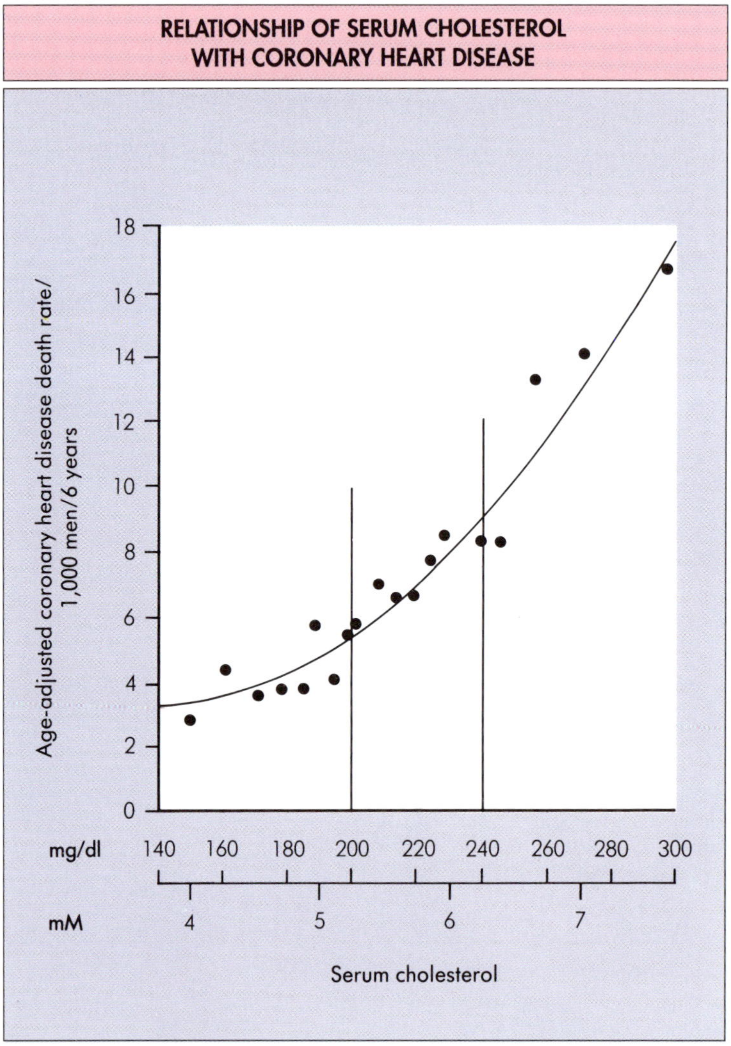

Fig. 4.10 The Multiple Risk Factor Intervention Trial: Relationship between levels of serum cholesterol and risks of fatal coronary artery disease in a longitudinal study of more than 361,000 men screened for entry into the trial. Data modified from Stamler J, Wentworth D, Neaton JD. *J Am Med Assoc* 1986;**256**:2823.

Changes in Mortality Rates

CHANGES IN MORTALITY RATES FROM ISCHAEMIC HEART DISEASE

Over the period of 1968–1985, there have been dramatic changes in the pattern of ischaemic heart disease, with the incidence in males in the USA falling by approximately 20%, the rates in the UK remaining almost constant (Fig. 4.11), and the rates in Japan remaining at a uniformly low level.

The causes for the reduction in mortality rate in the USA are unclear. This fall may be due to National Education programmes which have led to a greater awareness of the problem, and to an active desire of the population to treat the known risk factors such as hypertension, hyperlipidaemia, smoking, and obesity. From this viewpoint, the

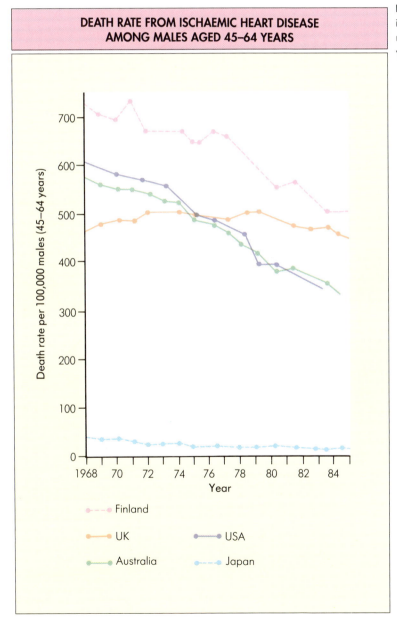

Fig. 4.11 Death rate due to ischaemic heart disease amongst males, aged 45–64, between the years 1968–85.

Epidemiology of Blood Lipids and Atherosclerosis

UK population would be regarded as indifferent or disinterested in the problem of the prevention of ischaemic heart disease. The death rates in women, although much lower than men, follow the same general trends, with falling rates in the USA and Australia, but fairly constant rates in the UK (Fig. 4.12).

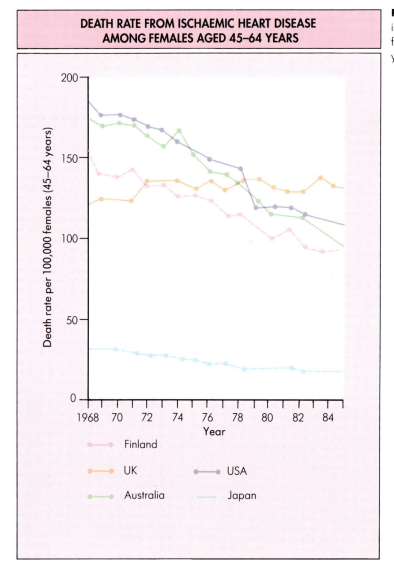

Fig. 4.12 Death rate due to ischaemic heart disease amongst females, aged 45–64, between the years 1968–85.

CHAPTER FIVE

Complications of Hyperlipidaemia

THE EYELIDS

Raised levels of blood lipids often give rise to ectopic lipid deposits in the skin, tendons, and eyes. The deposits in the eyelids (xanthelasma) usually accumulate near the inner canthus (Fig. 5.1), but as they enlarge, they can spread around the orbit of the eye (Fig. 5.2). The deposits are frequently noticed by ophthalmologists who excise them for cosmetic reasons. If, however, the

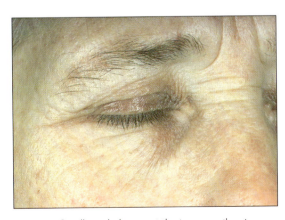

Fig. 5.1 Small xanthelasma at the inner canthus in a patient with Familial Hypercholesterolaemia.

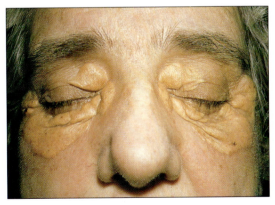

Fig. 5.2 Gross xanthelasma which have spread around the orbit of the eye in a patient with Familial Hypercholesterolaemia.

Complications of Hyperlipidaemia

underlying hyperlipidaemia remains untreated, the deposits usually re-accumulate (Fig. 5.3). Furthermore, a valuable chance to initiate therapy may be lost.

Although the deposits around the eyelids may have no adverse affects, their presence indicates that blood lipids should be measured. It is not yet clear why lipids have a tendency to deposit in the eyelids, but it may be due to the existence of a peculiarity in the permeability of the blood vessels in this region, or to the fact that connective-tissue proteins in this area may avidly bind extravascular lipoproteins. Occasionally, gross lipid deposits occur in the eyelids of subjects with entirely normal levels of blood lipids, suggesting that local tissue factors must play a predominant role.

If the underlying hyperlipidaemia is actively treated, xanthelasma often regresses, thereby providing encouraging evidence for the patient that treatment is beneficial.

SKIN AND TENDONS

Patients with Familial Hypercholesterolaemia often develop lipid deposits over the extensor surfaces of the elbows, knees, ankles, and hands. The cause is unclear but it is possible that repetitive trauma may cause the blood vessels at these sites to become more permeable and thus allow extravasation of circulating lipoproteins into the extravascular space.

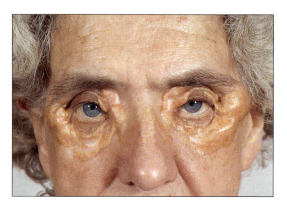

Fig. 5.3 Scarring of the periorbital skin and re-accumulation of xanthelasma after previous surgical excision.

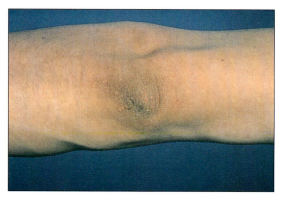

Fig. 5.4 Eruptive xanthomata over the elbow of a patient with mild hypertriglyceridaemia.

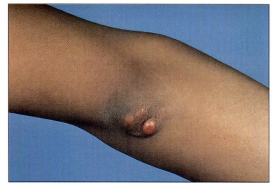

Fig. 5.5 Xanthomata over the elbow of a patient with severe hypertriglyceridaemia.

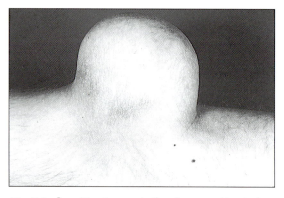

Fig. 5.6 Repetitive trauma to the elbow resulting in the formation of gross tendon xanthomata.

Deposits of lipids on the elbow can be quite difficult to see, and careful examination is required in order to detect them (Fig. 5.4). The deposits are easier to see in patients with more severe hypertriglyceridaemia (Fig. 5.5), and are characteristic of eruptive xanthomata. Occasionally, the deposits in the elbow can be quite large (Fig. 5.6).

The Achilles tendon is a common site for the accumulation of lipids. Accumulation can be so extensive (Fig. 5.7) that it can cause a rupture of the tendon on the slightest traumata. Spontaneous rupture of the Achilles tendon can indeed be the initial presenting feature of Familial Hypercholesterolaemia.

Deposits of lipids in the hands can resemble gout, as was the case of the patient shown in Fig. 5.8, who was initially referred to a rheumatologist. The patient was eventually found to have Familial Hypercholesterolaemia. More usually, the deposits in the tendons of the hands are less noticeable (Fig. 5.9). Infiltration of lipids in the tendons of the hand does not generally give rise to adverse functional effects, and can be quite minimal in appearance (Fig. 5.10). The deposits need to be actively sought in suspected cases of Familial Hypercholesterolaemia.

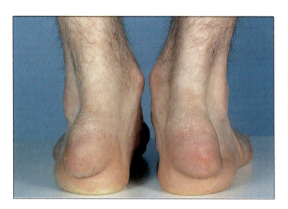

Fig. 5.7 Extensive accumulation of lipids in the Achilles tendon in a patient with Familial Hypercholesterolaemia.

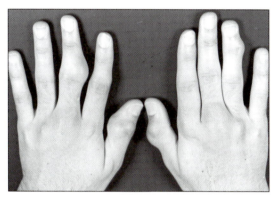

Fig. 5.8 Gross deformities of the hand due to tendon xanthomata in a patient with Familial Hypercholesterolaemia.

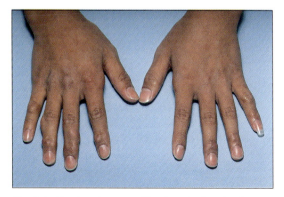

Fig. 5.9 Tendon deposits of lipids in the hands of a young girl with hypercholesterolaemia.

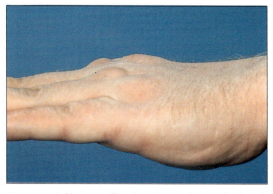

Fig. 5.10 Infiltration of lipids in the tendons of the hand. Careful palpation of the knuckles is required in order to detect these small xanthomata.

Complications of Hyperlipidaemia

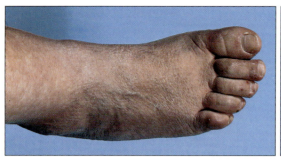
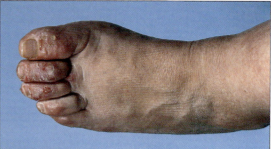

Fig. 5.11 Deformities of the tendons of the feet due to deposition of cholesterol. Surgical correction is occasionally required.

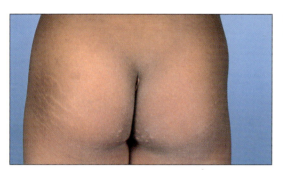

Fig. 5.12 Deposit of lipids over the buttocks of a child with heterozygous Familial Hypercholesterolaemia.

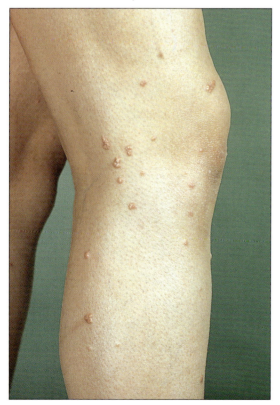

Fig. 5.13 Crops of eruptive xanthomata in a patient with alcoholic hypertriglyceridaemia.

Deposits over the feet can give rise to gross functional disabilities as seen in the patient in Fig. 5.11. This patient required major orthopaedic surgery to correct gross tendon deformities in her feet, which were due to extensive cholesterol deposits.

Deposits of lipids are also commonly found over the buttocks, as seen in the child with heterozygous Familial Hypercholesterolaemia in Fig. 5.12.

In severe hypertriglyceridaemia, the pattern of cutaneous lipid deposition is very different, and ectopic deposits of lipids can occur anywhere over the skin surface. Eruptive xanthomata can occur in patients with severe hypertriglyceridaemia from any cause (Fig. 5.13). These deposits usually disappear rapidly when the hyperlipidaemia is treated.

Complications of Hyperlipidaemia in the Eye

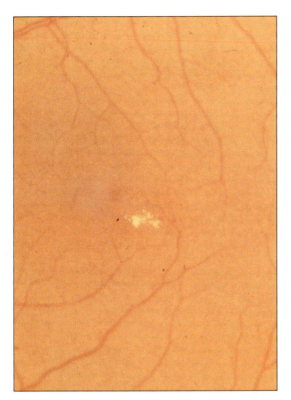

Fig. 6.3 Probable retinal xanthoma in a patient with polygenic hypertriglyceridaemia.

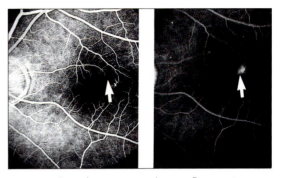

Fig. 6.4 Retinal angiograms showing fluorescein trapped in retinal deposits.

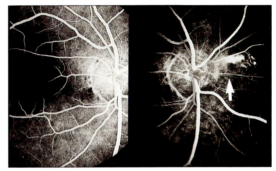

Fig. 6.5 Fluorescein angiograms of a patient with hypertriglyceridaemia, showing a retinal leak.

retinal angiogram of the eye, after an intravenous injection of fluorescein, shows that fluorescein leaks into the retinal deposit (Fig. 6.4). The lesion would be expected to resolve on treatment of the hyperlipidaemia. Retinal leaks of fluorescein are the most common effects of severe hyperlipidaemia (Fig. 6.5). It is not yet clear why retinal vascular permeability increases in severe hyperlipidaemia, but an associated hypertension would be expected to exacerbate the condition.

The venous thrombotic effects of hyperlipidaemia are more serious, and less-well recognized. Recurrent attacks of acute pancreatitis occur in severe hypertriglyceridaemia, these probably being due to a predisposition to venous thrombosis which favours leakage of exocrine pancreatic enzymes and initiates pancreatic damage. The aetiological steps which may be involved in venous thrombosis are shown in Fig. 6.6. Blood lipids interact with the membrane of the platelet, thus affecting the release of its stored granules (Fig.

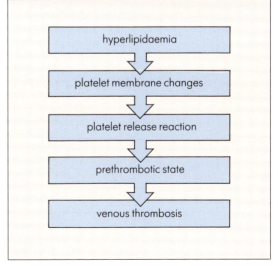

Fig. 6.6 Possible aetiological steps involved in venous thrombosis.

6.7). These granules contain β-thromboglobulin, platelet factor 4, and other pro-coagulant materials. All these components are found at elevated concentrations in the plasma of hyperlipidaemic subjects (Fig. 6.8). The increase in malondialdehyde formation in the platelets from patients with hyperlipidaemia is a reflection of the activation of the prostaglandin pathways of metabolism (Fig. 6.9). The

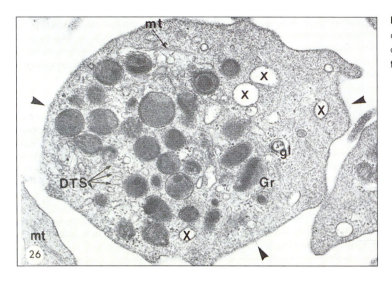

Fig. 6.7 An electron micrograph of a platelet showing storage granules of pro-coagulant materials (β-thromboglobulin, platelet factor 4).

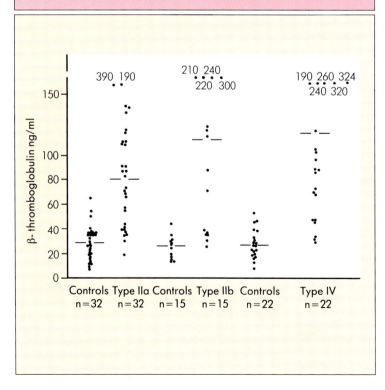

Fig. 6.8 Platelet function in hyperlipidaemia: Mean and range of plasma β-thromboglobulin (ng/ml) of 69 patients with three types of hyperlipidaemia, and of age- and sex-matched controls. The difference (Student's unpaired t test) between the mean logarithmic values in patients with each type of hyperlipidaemia and controls was highly significant ($p<0.001$). Data modified from Zahavi J, Betteridge JD, Galton DJ, Kakkar VV. *Am J Med* 1981;**70**:59.

result is a predisposition to platelet aggregation and to intravascular thrombosis, which in the eye, can give rise to retinal vessel occlusion. A study which was conducted at the Moorfields Eye Hospital showed that hypertension, diabetes, and hyperlipidaemia, were the most frequently seen associations with retinal vascular thrombosis (Fig. 6.10).

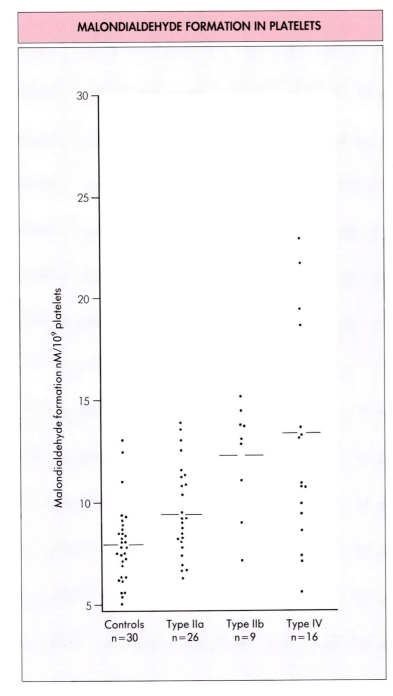

Fig. 6.9 Malondialdehyde formation in platelets. Mean and range of malondialdehyde formation (nmol/10^9 platelets) in washed platelets of 51 patients with three types of hyperlipidaemia and of 30 controls. The difference (Student's unpaired *t* test) between the mean values of patients and controls was highly significant ($p<0.001$ in patients with Type IIb and Type IV hyperlipidaemia, and $p<0.014$ in patients with Type IIa hyperlipidaemia). Data modified from Zahavi J, Betteridge JD, Galton DJ, Kakkar VV. *Am J Med* 1981;**70**:59.

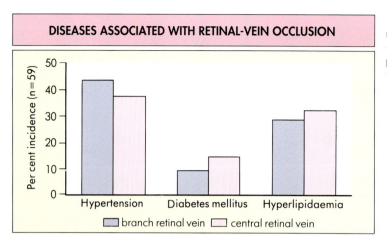

Fig. 6.10 Diseases associated with retinal-vein occlusion. Data modified from Dodson PM, Galton DJ, Hamilton AM, Black RK. *Brit J Ophth* 1982;**66**:161.

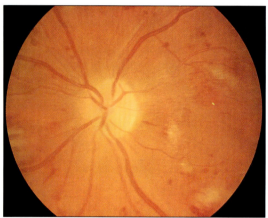

Fig. 6.11 Central retinal-vein occlusion in a patient with hyperlipidaemia as the only observed pathogenic factor.

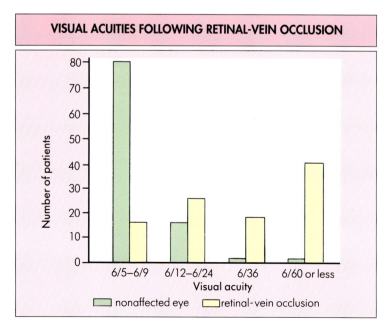

Fig. 6.12 Visual acuities following retinal-vein occlusion compared to acuity in the unaffected eye in 99 patients. Data modified from Dodson PM, Galton DJ, Hamilton AM, Black RK. *Brit J Ophth* 1982;**66**:161.

Complications of Hyperlipidaemia in the Eye

A central-vein occlusion is recognized by the presence of a ring of haemorrhages and exudates which occur around the optic disc, and of prominently congested retinal veins (Fig. 6.11). The visual acuity in such conditions can fall below 6/60 on the Snellen chart (Fig. 6.12). Branch retinal-vein occlusions, such as inferior hemisphere retinal-vein occlusion, are more common (Fig. 6.13). The disturbance of the retinal vasculature in this region causes a scotoma which can resolve depending on the extent of the local vessel closure and the later formation of collateral vessels. Peripheral vascular closure can also occur in, for example, an inferior temporal retinal-vein thrombosis (Fig. 6.14). Another example of vessel closure in an inferior hemisphere retinal-vein occlusion is shown in Fig. 6.15. The ischaemic areas can provoke the formation of new vessels (Fig. 6.16), which occasionally requires treatment by photocoagulation.

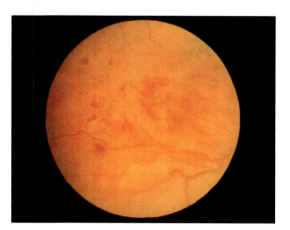

Fig. 6.13 A branch retinal-vein occlusion in a patient with hyperlipidaemia as the only pathogenic factor.

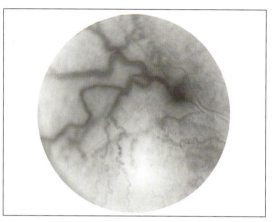

Fig. 6.14 A fluorescein angiogram of an inferior temporal retinal-vein occlusion showing peripheral vessel closure in a patient with hyperlipidaemia. The relative avascular area at approximately 4–6 o'clock is clearly apparent.

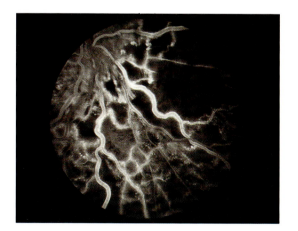

Fig. 6.15 Peripheral vessel closure of an inferior hemisphere retinal-vein occlusion in a patient with hyperlipidaemia. The avascular area is seen at 12–3 o'clock.

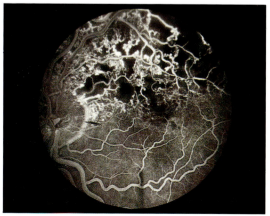

Fig. 6.16 Formation of new vessels in the inferior hemisphere territory following retinal-vein thrombosis, in a patient with hyperlipidaemia.

Elevated plasma levels of both platelet factor 4 (Fig. 6.17) and β-thromboglobulin (Fig. 6.18) can be found in patients with retinal-vein occlusion, and these may contribute to the thrombotic process. The visual acuities in the affected eyes commonly fall to below 6/9; the acuities fall to 6/60 or less only in central venous occlusion (see *Fig. 6.12*). In the elderly, a fall in acuity can produce troublesome visual disability, and hence severe hyperlipidaemia should be treated even in this age group. Although hypolipidaemic therapy may not affect the prognosis for atherosclerotic

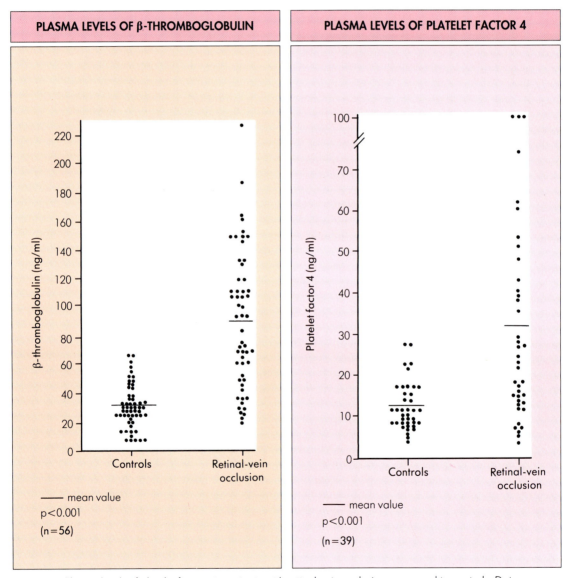

Fig. 6.17 Plasma levels of platelet factors in patients with retinal-vein occlusion compared to controls. Data modified from Dodson PM, Westwick J, Kakkar VV, Galton DJ. *Brit J Ophth* 1983;**67**:143.

complications, it may help to prevent retinal vascular accidents. When the formation of new vessels is stimulated after retinal-vein thrombosis, the patient may sometimes require photocoagulation, using a laser beam, to preserve the macular area, the aim being to destroy the leash of new vessels that encroach on the macular region (Fig. 6.19). Alternatively, photocoagulation may be required to prevent neovascular (haemorrhagic) glaucoma which develops after central retinal-vein thrombosis.

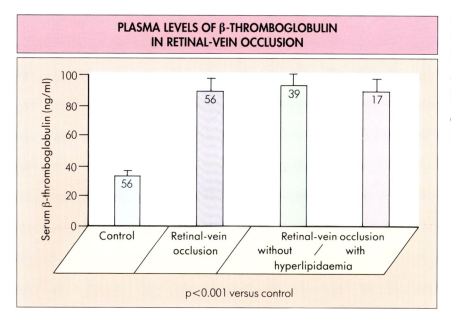

Fig. 6.18 Plasma levels of β-thromboglobulin in patients with retinal-vein occlusion compared to controls. Data modified from Dodson PM, Westwick J, Kakkar VV, Galton DJ. *Brit J Ophth* 1983;**67**:143.

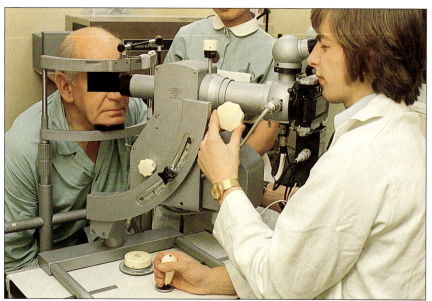

Fig. 6.19 A patient undergoing photocoagulation to treat new vessel formation following retinal-vein occlusion. This is carried out particularly if the macular region is threatened.

Complications of Hyperlipidaemia in the Eye

CASE REPORT

A patient presented with headaches which were becoming worse, nausea, bilateral papilloedema, and nystagmus on right lateral gaze. Large xanthomata were noted on the elbows, knees, and Achilles tendon (Fig. 6.20). An X-ray of the skull revealed a lesion which was invading the right posterior fossa (Fig. 6.21). A CAT scan showed dilated ventricles with a large space-occupying lesion in the right middle and posterior fossae (Fig. 6.22). Craniotomy was performed and a large extradural mass was excised. Histological examination showed this mass to be a large cholesterol xanthoma which had numerous cholesterol clefts surrounded by foamy macrophages (Fig. 6.23). Blood levels of cholesterol were found to be 18mM (696mg/dl) and those of triglycerides, 10mM (886mg/dl). Analysis of serum lipoproteins by density-gradient centrifugation showed increased concentrations of both LDL and VLDL. The family tree of the patient revealed that there was a dominant inheritance of Familial Combined Hyperlipidaemia (Fig. 6.24). The response to treatment with cholestyramine and bezafibrate was dramatic, persistent normolipidaemia being achieved with the aim of preventing recurrence of

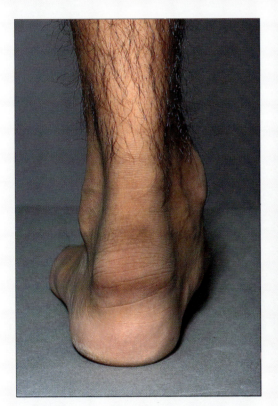

Fig. 6.20 Large xanthomata on the Achilles tendon of the patient.

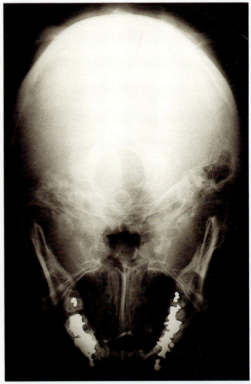

Fig. 6.21 An X-ray of the skull revealing a lesion which is invading the right posterior fossa.

intracranial xanthoma. Xanthomata can occur potentially at any tissue site, although intracranial lesions are rare. There was perhaps some predisposing feature present in this patient, such as a small arteriovenous malformation, which favoured the accumulation of lipid in the posterior fossa.

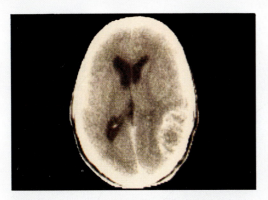

Fig. 6.22 A CAT scan showing dilated ventricles and a large space-occupying lesion in the right middle and posterior fossae.

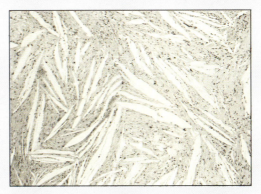

Fig. 6.23 Histology of large intracranial xanthoma showing numerous cholesterol clefts and foam cells. Courtesy of Rees A, Lee G, Stocks J, Vella MA, Galton DJ. *Brit Med J* 1984;**288**:1722.

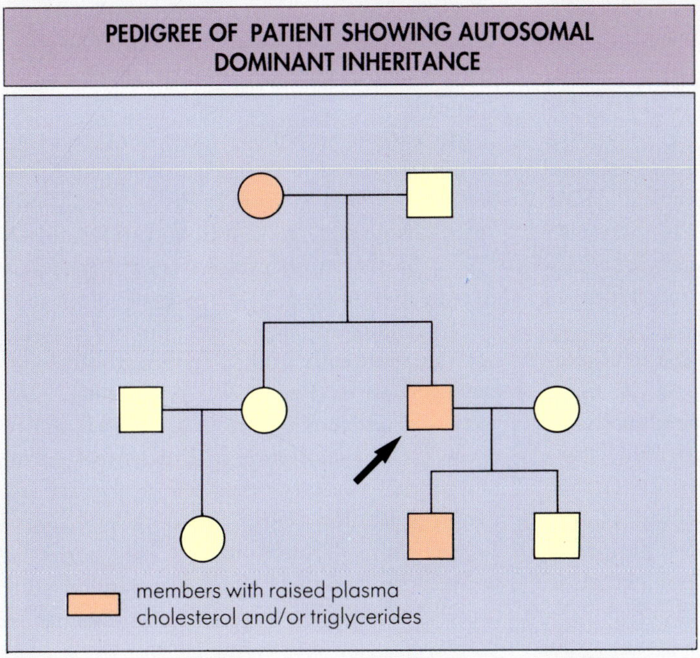

Fig. 6.24 Pedigree of the patient showing autosomal dominant inheritance of Familial Combined Hyperlipidaemia.

CHAPTER SEVEN

Complications of Hyperlipidaemia at the Arterial Wall

Premature atherosclerosis is a major complication of hyperlipidaemia. Prevention or regression of atheroma is as much an aim of treatment of hyperlipidaemia as is the reduction of the levels of fats in the blood. The main atherogenic hyperlipidaemias are Familial Hypercholesterolaemia (Type IIa), Familial Dysbetalipoproteinaemia (Type III), Familial Combined Hypertriglyceridaemia, and Familial Hypertriglyceridaemia with low HDL. Familial Chylomicronaemia (Type I) is not usually associated with atheroma. The size of chylomicrons probably exclude their entry into the subendothelial space.

Multiple aetiological routes can lead to atherosclerosis. Single gene defects, such as the LDL-receptor mutation in Familial Hypercholesterolaemia, polygenic defects, such as Familial Dysbetalipoproteinaemia, and environmental factors, such as smoking and high dietary intake of fat, can all predispose an individual to develop premature atherosclerosis. Other factors can also be involved in the pathogenesis of atherosclerosis (Fig. 7.1). However, the distinction between genetic and environmental factors cannot always be easily made. Some diseases, for example, diabetes mellitus, are affected by environmental factors, but they also have strong genetic determinants. Many other disorders require an interplay of genetic and environmental factors before the disease becomes manifest.

The early lesion of atheroma can be recognized by small areas of fatty streaks which consist of an accumulation of fat-laden cells in the subintimal space. These provoke a mild fibrous reaction (Fig. 7.2a). As the lesion progresses, the arterial wall becomes damaged, with the development of irregular intimal plaques and a loss of endothelial surface, eventually leading to thrombosis over the damaged areas (Fig. 7.2b). A close-up view of fatty streaks at the root of the aorta (Fig. 7.3) show their co-existence with extensive coronary atherosclerosis, producing left ventricular myocardial infarction (Fig. 7.4). Both early and late lesions have been found in the same individual, simultaneously, and this patient with an unusual form of hypercholesterolaemia, died of myocardial infarction in the third decade (Fig. 7.4).

Complications of Hyperlipidaemia at the Arterial Wall

INTERACTION BETWEEN ENVIRONMENTAL AND GENETIC FACTORS

Genetic factors	Environmental factors

lipoprotein abnormalities
  LDL-receptor
  apolipoproteins
 	
clotting disturbances
 	
vessel wall
  fibronectin
  glycosaminoglycans
 	
smooth-muscle proliferation
  platelet-derived growth factor
  epidermal growth factor
  insulin/insulin receptor
	diet
	
	smoking
	
	secondary to other associated disease, for example, diabetes mellitus
	
	stress
	
	exercise

hypertension	

Fig. 7.1 The complex interaction amongst environmental and genetic factors involved in the pathogenesis of atheroma.

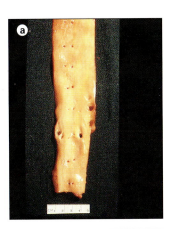

Fig. 7.2 An arterial wall affected with (a) minimal atheroma (fatty streaks) and (b) severe atheroma.

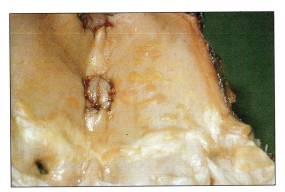

Fig. 7.3 A close-up view of fatty streaks in the root of the aorta in a patient with Familial Hypercholesterolaemia.

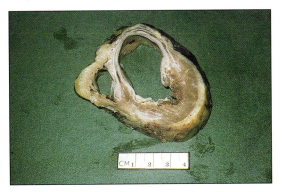

Fig. 7.4 Myocardial infarction, the end result of severe coronary atherosclerosis where the myocardium is reduced to a rim of scar tissue.

The arterial trees which are commonly affected by atherosclerosis to produce clinical features are the coronary (Fig. 7.5), peripheral (iliac, femoral) (Fig. 7.6), and carotid/cerebral vessels (Fig. 7.7), since they all tend to have a poor collateral circulation.

Complications of Hyperlipidaemia at the Arterial Wall

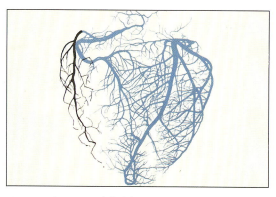

Fig. 7.5 A wax model of the arterial supply to the heart with obstruction to one branch (in black) showing the poor collateral circulation of its territory.

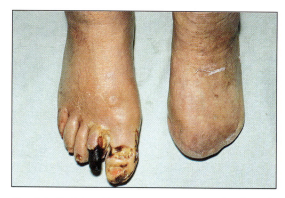

Fig. 7.6 Peripheral leg arteries are commonly affected by atherosclerosis.

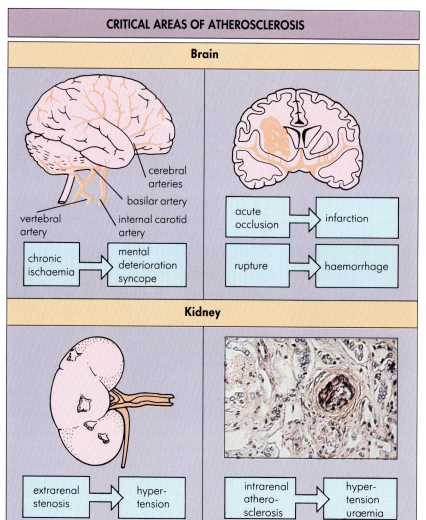

Fig. 7.7 The carotid and intracranial cerebral vessels are often affected by atherosclerosis.

DEVELOPMENT OF ATHEROMA

The early lesion of atheroma (the fatty streak) is due to the accumulation of fat-laden (foam) cells, in the subendothelial space. These foam cells are derived mainly from circulating monocytes which are filled with phagocytosed lipid (from circulating lipoproteins) (Figs. 7.8 and 7.9). The development of the fatty streak involves foam cells from the circulation moving into the early arterial-wall lesion, possibly because of damage to the endothelial surface lining (Fig. 7.10). Smooth-muscle

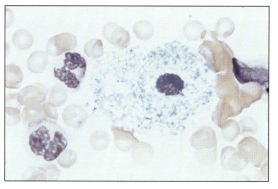

Fig. 7.8 A circulating monocyte which has transformed into a foam cell in a patient with hyperlipidaemia. Aggregation of such foam cells in the subintimal space initiates the development of the fatty streak.

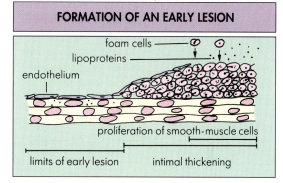

Fig. 7.9 A scheme for the development of the fatty streak, showing the origin of foam cells.

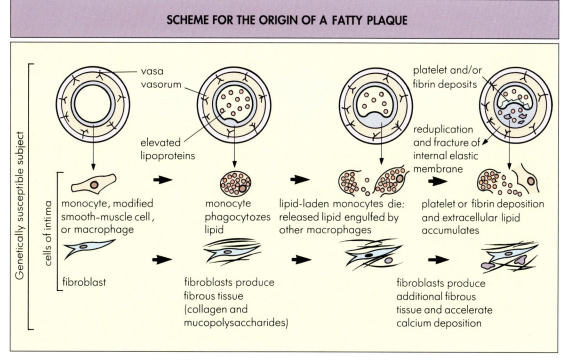

Fig. 7.10 A scheme for the origin of the fatty plaque, showing how foam cells derived from circulating monocytes, and proliferation of smooth-muscle cells cause a raised arterial fibro-fatty plaque.

cells proliferate, move into the early plaque, and either lay down collagen to form a fibrous plaque, or they may round-up to become foam cells as they accumulate lipid (Fig. 7.10).

As the lesion progresses, the fatty streak enlarges, accumulates extracellular lipid, and provokes a fibrous reaction (somewhat analogous to wound healing after tissue damage) (Fig. 7.11). This leads to the development of an elevated fibro-fatty plaque with a denuded endothelial lining that predisposes to platelet aggregation, fibrin deposition, and at some sites, to an intravascular thrombosis which causes a clinical event (myocardial or cerebral infarction).

The earliest stage at which therapy should be directed is when foam cells are formed from modified lipoprotein particles, and when damage to the endothelial-cell barrier (by hypertension or smoking) allows foam cells to penetrate and accumulate in the subintimal space. Raised levels of circulating lipid in the bloodstream will favour the formation and accumulation of foam cells in the arterial wall, as well as at other tissue sites; the formation of foam cells is the main reason for the treatment of hyperlipidaemia.

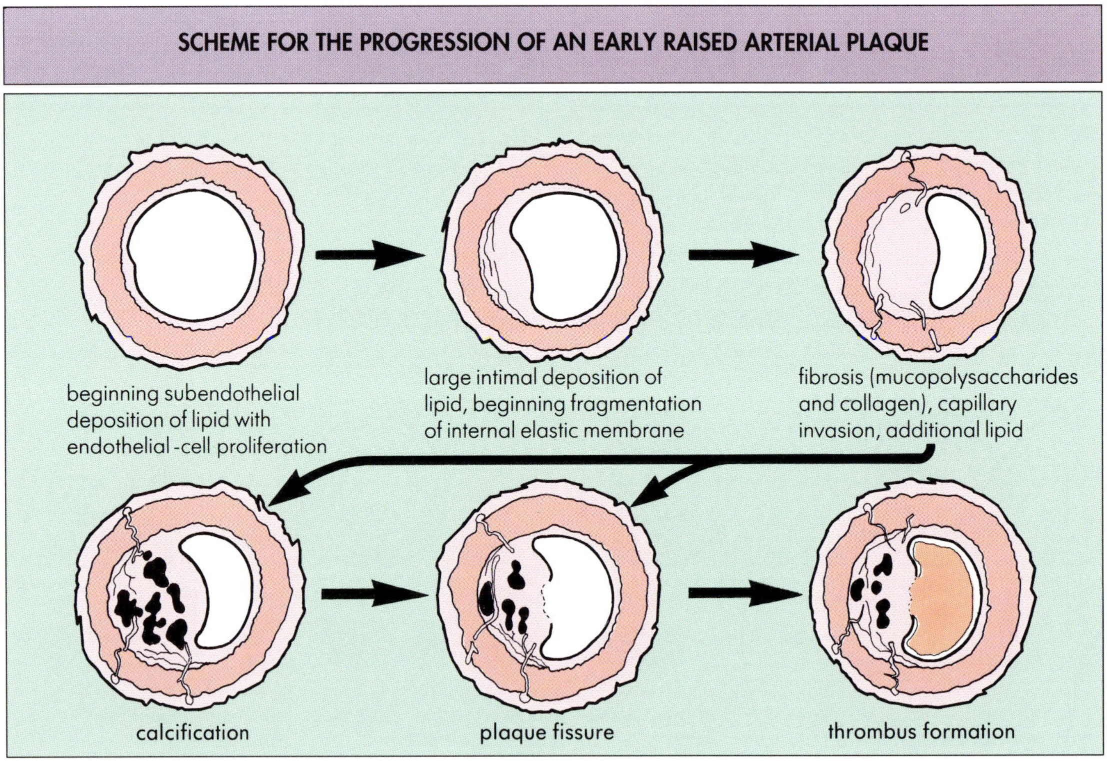

SCHEME FOR THE PROGRESSION OF AN EARLY RAISED ARTERIAL PLAQUE

- beginning subendothelial deposition of lipid with endothelial-cell proliferation
- large intimal deposition of lipid, beginning fragmentation of internal elastic membrane
- fibrosis (mucopolysaccharides and collagen), capillary invasion, additional lipid
- calcification
- plaque fissure
- thrombus formation

Fig. 7.11 A scheme for the progression of the early raised arterial plaque, showing fibrosis, enlargement, fibrin deposition, occasionally calcification, and eventually fissure and thrombosis, on the wall of the plaque.

DETECTION OF ATHEROMA

Effective means of preventing atheroma initially require reliable techniques for its early detection and progression (or regression) after therapeutic intervention.

Invasive techniques

Angiography

Angiography is the standard method currently used to assess the extent and severity of atherosclerosis, particularly in the coronary vessels (Fig.

Detection of Atheroma

7.12). Differential subtraction angiography (DSA) is less invasive in that a small amount of radio-contrast material is injected intravenously, to image the arterial wall. The method of DSA is more costly than angiography, due to the use of high-quality image intensifiers and video-camera recording to visualize the major arterial vessels. Images obtained prior to the arrival of the radio-contrast material are subtracted electronically from the subsequent images to reveal only the vascular tree.

Noninvasive techniques

Doppler ultrasound

In Doppler ultrasound, a beam of ultrasound is reflected off red cells which are moving in the arterial lumen. The interference pattern of the reflected sound waves varies according to the speed and turbulence of flow produced by arterial-wall disease or obstruction (Fig. 7.13). This method is particularly useful for the detection of atheroma in arteries which are easily accessible, such as the

Fig. 7.12 An angiogram showing gross irregularity and obstruction of the coronary artery.

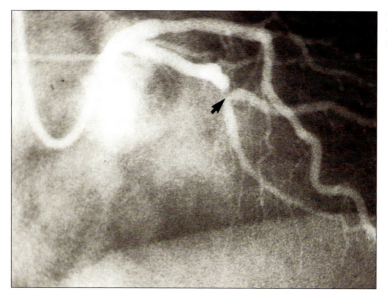

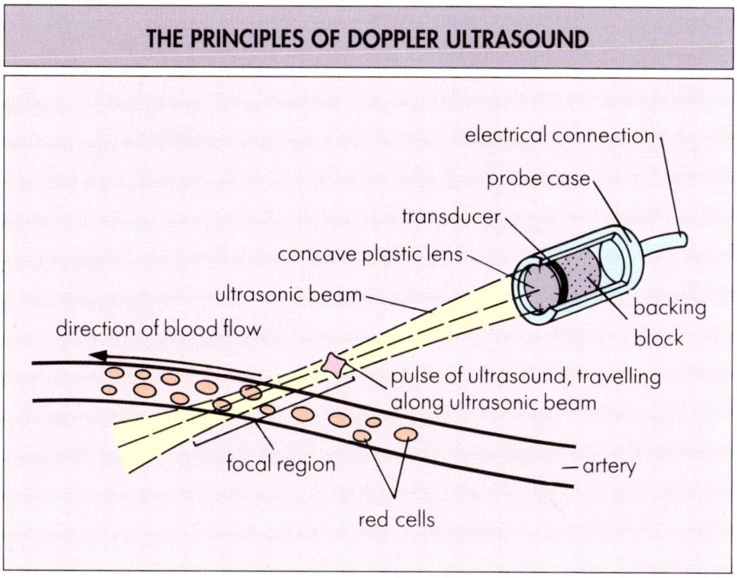

Fig. 7.13 The principles of Doppler ultrasound. A pulse of ultrasound is generated by the probe and is weakly focused onto the blood vessel. Reflection of sound waves from red cells affects the pulse-echo waveform.

Complications of Hyperlipidaemia at the Arterial Wall

carotids or femorals. A typical instrument which is used for the examination of the major arteries is shown in Fig. 7.14. Waveforms produced from obstructed and patent femoral arteries are shown in Fig. 7.15. When the artery is obstructed by more than 50%, there is no reverse flow during diastole, and the waveform is blunted (Fig. 7.16).

Magnetic resonance imaging

The principle used in magnetic resonance imaging is based on radio waves emitted from protons when resonated in a magnetic field (Fig. 7.17).

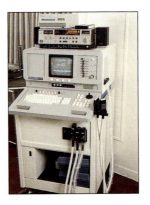

Fig. 7.14 Typical Doppler-ultrasound equipment used for the examination of the major arteries.

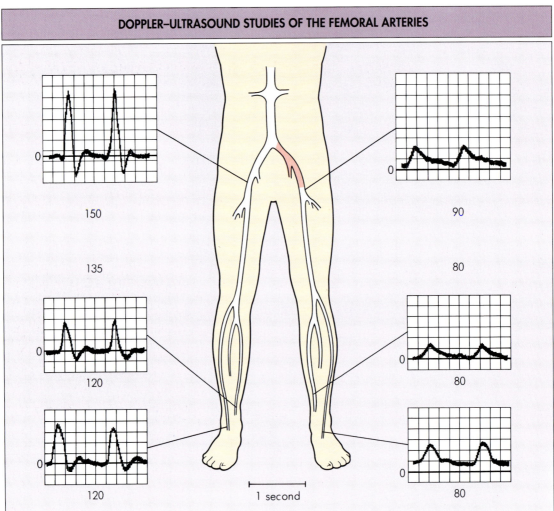

Fig. 7.15 The arrangement for Doppler-ultrasound studies of the femoral arteries, and a schematic view of the results. Note the differences in waveform obtained from a patient with an obstructed femoral artery.

Detection of Atheroma

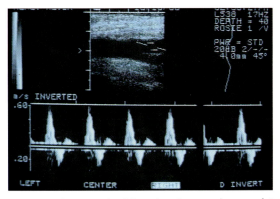
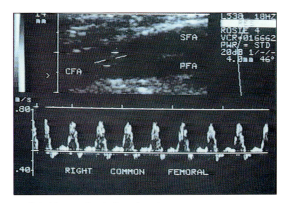

Fig. 7.16 An example of Doppler-ultrasound scans of the superficial femoral arteries, showing obstruction in the right vessel (absence of reverse flow, and a plaque visible in the lumen of the artery).

THE PRINCIPLES OF MAGNETIC RESONANCE IMAGING

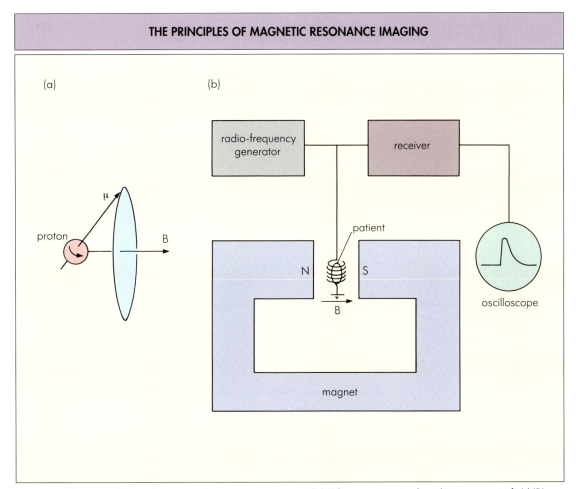

Fig. 7.17 The principles used in magnetic resonance imaging. (a) When a proton is placed in a magnetic field (B), the magnetic moment precesses around the direction of the field. Application of the resonant radio-frequency pulse affects the magnetization, depending on the locality of the protons. (b) A schematic arrangement for detecting nuclear magnetic resonance from protons.

The location of protons in an aqueous or non-aqueous environment will affect the emitted signals, and since atheroma is a water-excluding area, it should theoretically resolve well by magnetic resonance. Images can be produced which clearly show the site of the carotid-artery obstruction.

At present, magnetic-resonance scans take a long time to perform, and the resolution is often inferior to that of angiography. If sufficient technical advances occur to overcome these obstacles, the technique may displace the more complicated and invasive methods of angiography.

CHAPTER EIGHT
Secondary Hyperlipidaemias

Many common systemic diseases, such as diabetes mellitus, obesity, and alcohol abuse, can give rise to a secondary hyperlipidaemia (Fig. 8.1). These diseases should be excluded before treating a lipid

SOME CAUSES OF SECONDARY HYPERLIPIDAEMIA					
Condition	Main lipid abnormality	Chylo-microns	VLDL	LDL	HDL
Diabetes mellitus	↑ triglyceride	↑	↑	↑ or normal	↓
Alcohol abuse	↑ triglyceride	↑	↑		↓
Drugs, for example, steroids, thiazides, β-blockers	↑ triglyceride and/or ↑ cholesterol		↑	↑	
Hypothyroidism	↑ cholesterol			↑	
Chronic renal failure	↑ triglyceride		↑	↑ or normal	
Nephrotic syndrome	↑ cholesterol and ↑ triglyceride		↑	↑	
Cholestasis	↑ cholesterol			↑	↓
Obesity	↑ triglyceride	↑	↑		↓

Fig. 8.1 Some causes of secondary hyperlipidaemia.

Secondary Hyperlipidaemias

disorder; for example, patients with hypercholesterolaemia should initially be tested for hypothyroidism before commencing treatment (Fig. 8.2). However, in some particularly common disorders, such as diabetes mellitus, treatment of the underlying condition may not affect the lipaemia, and it is then assumed that two primary conditions (diabetes and lipaemia) co-exist and require separate treatments.

DIABETES MELLITUS

Diabetes mellitus is considered to be a disorder of glucose metabolism, but insulin also has a profound effect on protein and lipid metabolism. Disturbances of lipid homeostasis always occur in untreated or poorly controlled Type I insulin-dependent diabetes mellitus (IDDM) or Type II noninsulin-dependent diabetes mellitus (NIDDM). The disturbances of lipid metabolism may well account for the major complications and cause of death of diabetics due to atherosclerotic lesions in the coronary, cerebral, and peripheral arterial trees

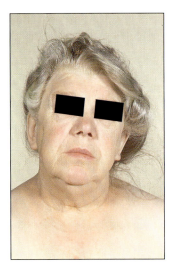

Fig. 8.2 A patient with mild hypercholesterolaemia who was shown subsequently to have hypothyroidism.

(Fig. 8.3). Severe diabetic lipaemia is characteristic of the electrophoretic pattern of Fredrickson Type V (Fig. 8.4), and diabetics with hyperlipidaemia are more likely to have arterial-wall disease than those with normal plasma lipids (Fig. 8.5). More than 50% of diabetic women and men with proven atheroma have hyperlipidaemia (Fig. 8.6). In both

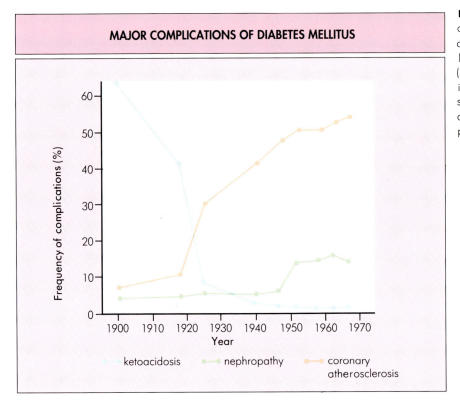

Fig. 8.3 The major complication of diabetes mellitus is no longer the comas (since the discovery of insulin), but atherosclerosis of the coronary, cerebral, and peripheral arteries.

PLASMA FEATURES OF TYPE V HYPERLIPIDAEMIA

Lipoprotein phenotype	Plasma cholesterol	Plasma triglyceride	Plasma appearance
Type V chylomicrons ↑↑ VLDL ↑↑↑	moderately elevated	markedly elevated	'cream-layer' over turbid to opaque infranatant

Fig. 8.4 Characteristic plasma features of diabetic lipaemia, Fredrickson Type V.

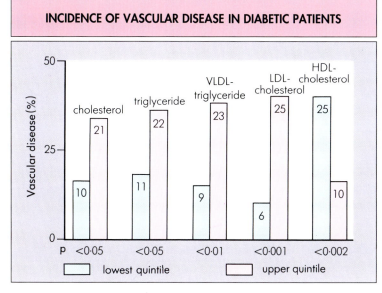

Fig. 8.5 A study at the lipid and diabetic clinics of St Bartholomew's Hospital, showing that patients in the upper quintiles of distribution for cholesterol, triglyceride, VLDL-triglyceride, and LDL-cholesterol, have more end points of vascular disease (infarct, angina, claudication, and ECG abnormalities) than patients in the lowest quintile. Data modified from Reckless JPD, Betteridge DJ, Wu P, Galton DJ. *Brit Med J* 1978;**i**:883.

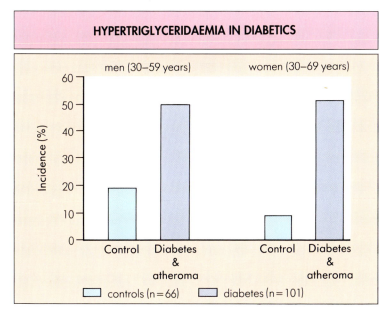

Fig. 8.6 The incidence of hyperlipidaemia in diabetic men and women with proven atheroma, compared to diabetics without atheroma. Data modified from Santen RJ, Willis PW, Fajans SS. *Arch Int Med* 1972;**130**:883.

insulin-deficient and insulin-resistant states, increased lipolysis occurs in adipose tissue, with either a raised plasma level, or flux of free fatty acids which is particularly seen overnight during the fasting state (Fig. 8.7).

The increased recycling of fatty acids to the liver, combined with hyperglycaemia, stimulates the synthesis of hepatic triglyceride and leads to Type IV hypertriglyceridaemia, the most common lipoprotein abnormality which occurs in poorly controlled diabetes mellitus (Fig. 8.8).

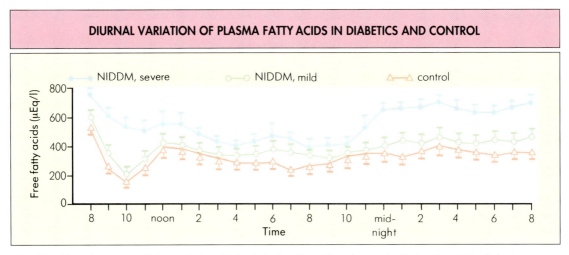

Fig. 8.7 Diurnal variation of plasma fatty acids in diabetics (Type II) and controls. During the night, diabetics run higher levels of fatty acids than controls. Data modified from Reaven GM, (personal communication).

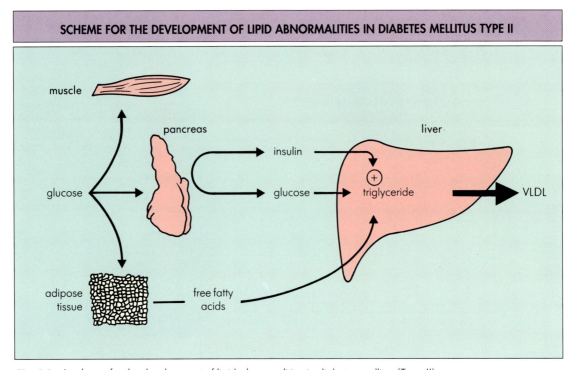

Fig. 8.8 A scheme for the development of lipid abnormalities in diabetes mellitus (Type II).

CASE REPORTS

Case 1

A man, aged 54, weighing 71kg, presented in 1975 with mild combined hyperlipidaemia. His levels of cholesterol were 8.2mM (317mg/dl) and of triglyceride, 3.6mM (319mg/dl) (Fig. 8.9). Random blood-glucose tests were normal at 3.6mM (64mg/dl), with a peak blood-glucose level of 8.8mM (158mg/dl) after a 50-g oral load. There was no family history of hyperlipidaemia or diabetes, and his weekly alcohol intake was less than 10 units. Lipid levels were stable between 1975–1979 using fibrates, and thereafter his levels of plasma triglyceride started to fluctuate between 8 and 22mM (708 and 1,967mg/dl); this was due to the development of diabetes mellitus with a rise in blood sugars of up to 20mM (360mg/dl) (Fig. 8.10).

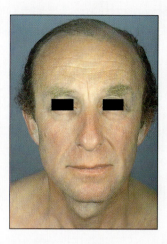

Fig. 8.9 A man, aged 54, with primary hyperlipidaemia which deteriorated when he developed diabetes mellitus (NIDDM).

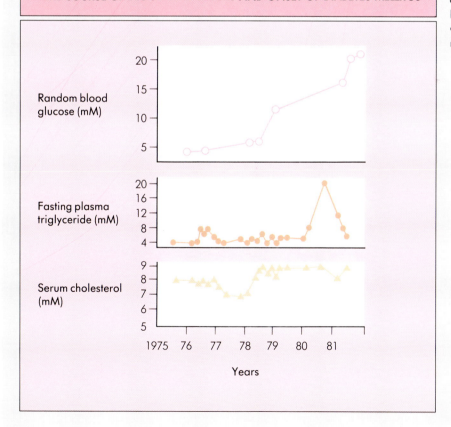

Fig. 8.10 Time course of blood lipid values, and onset of diabetes mellitus (NIDDM).

Case 2

A woman, aged 27, weighing 80kg, was found to have moderate hyperlipidaemia due to high levels of cholesterol, 8.8mM (341mg/dl) and triglyceride, 7.7mM (681mg/dl), which responded well to dietary measures; annual blood-glucose values were less than 7mM (126mg/dl). She then developed diabetes mellitus (Type II) with fasting blood-glucose values of 13mM (234mg/dl), and her lipid levels deteriorated grossly: triglycerides, 140mM (12.4g/dl); cholesterol, 42mM (1.6g/dl); this deterioration was associated with lipaemia retinalis, eruptive xanthomata (Fig. 8.11), and acute abdominal pain suggestive of pancreatitis. Treatment of her diabetes mellitus dramatically reduced the plasma levels of lipids, demonstrating the adverse effects of uncontrolled diabetes on levels of blood fats (Fig. 8.12).

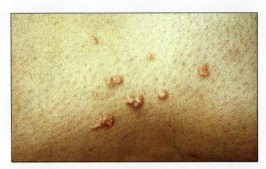

Fig. 8.11 Eruptive xanthomata on the skin of the patient with diabetic lipaemia.

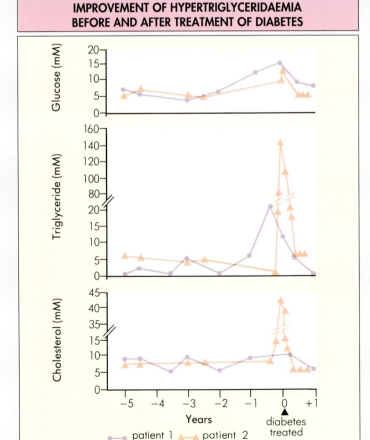

Fig. 8.12 Improvement in hyper-triglyceridaemia of two patients (Case 1 and Case 2) before and after treatment of their diabetes. Data modified from Thomas DJB, Stocks J, Galton DJ, Besser GM. *Diabetic Med* 1988;**5**:85.

Case 3

A woman, aged 37, weighing 69kg with severe diabetic lipaemia was treated with insulin. (Fig. 8.13). The clinical features of eruptive xanthomata, lipaemia retinalis, and acute pancreatitis, were similar to those observed in the patient described in *Case 2*, and although she did not require insulin for her diabetes, the levels of sugars in the blood, and of triglycerides, responded well to insulin therapy. Her state of insulin resistance protected her from any hypoglycaemic reactions with the doses of insulin which were administered, and was a useful form of hypolipidaemic therapy.

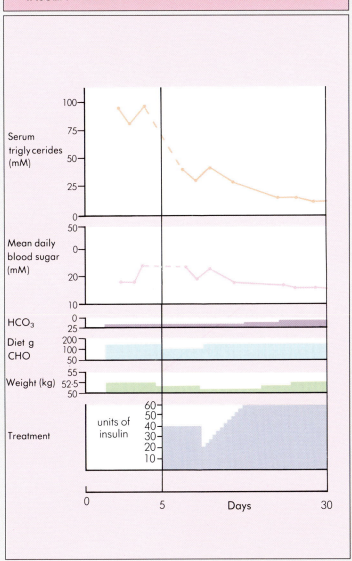

Fig. 8.13 The effect of insulin therapy on the levels of plasma triglycerides in the patient with diabetic lipaemia.

OBESITY

Caloric excess can lead not only to obesity (Fig. 8.14), but also to hypertriglyceridaemia in approximately 50% of cases. This may be partly due to the increased hepatic synthesis of lipoprotein-triglyceride for secretion and transport to adipose tissue for storage as fat. It is likely that the increased coronary morbidity and mortality associated with increasing body weight (Fig. 8.15) is due more to the circulating lipoprotein and hormonal abnormalities, than directly to the stored fat in the adipose organ.

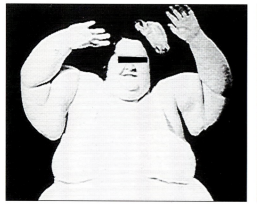
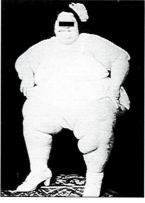
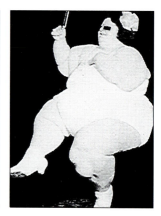

Fig. 8.14 An unusual case of obesity.

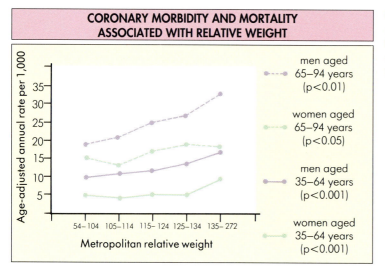

Fig. 8.15 Coronary morbidity and mortality, associated with increasing body weight, according to sex and weight. Data modified from Kannel WB. *Nutrition Rev* 1988;**46**:68.

ALCOHOLISM

Excessive alcohol consumption can also give rise to severe hyperlipidaemia. Although the causes are not clear, it is known that some of the biochemical features shown in Fig. 8.16 are involved. Metabolism of alcohol involves production of reduced pyridine nucleotides (NADH and NADPH from alcohol dehydrogenase) and this may stimulate the reductive synthesis of fatty acids in the liver from acetyl CoA and hence favour hepatic synthesis of triglyceride for secretion as VLDL.

Alcoholism

BIOCHEMICAL FACTORS THAT MAY LEAD TO ALCOHOLIC HYPERTRIGLYCERIDAEMIA

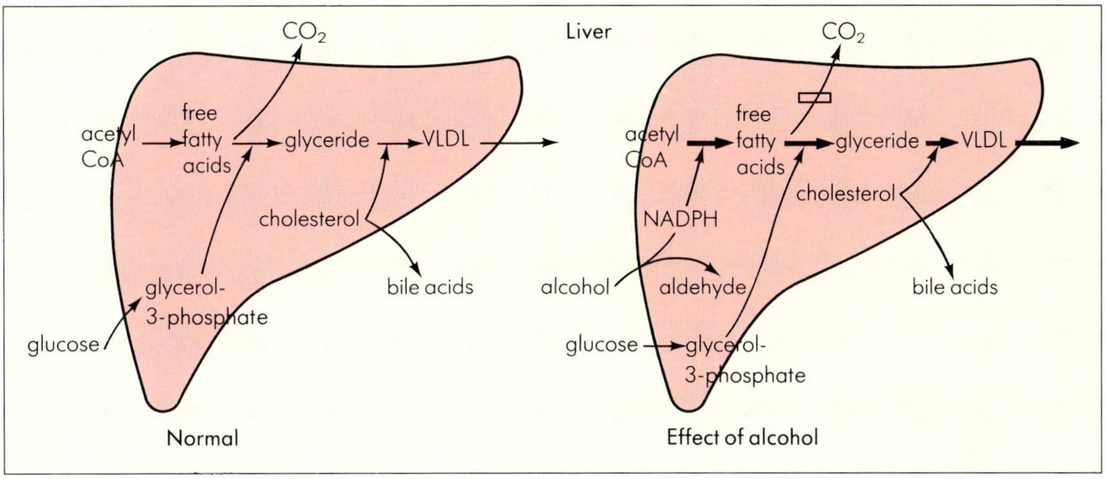

Fig. 8.16 Some biochemical factors that may lead to alcoholic hypertriglyceridaemia.

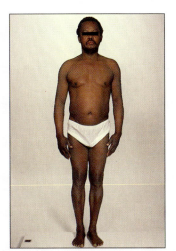

Fig. 8.17 A man, aged 48, who presented with severe alcoholic lipaemia.

CASE REPORT

A man, aged 48, presented with headaches and giddiness. Fasting plasma triglyceride levels were 95mM (8,404mg/dl), and cholesterol levels, 44mM (1,703mg/dl) (Fig.8.17). There were no associated arterial symptoms. He consumed from 7–10 pints of beer daily, and his intake increased considerably after news of his brother's death. Fundoscopy of the eye showed gross lipaemia retinalis (Fig. 8.18) with retinal-vessel closure in the periphery. During in-patient treatment, which comprised a zero-alcohol diet, his plasma lipid levels promptly fell to normal, and his liver-function tests improved (alkaline phosphatase levels fell from 120 to 84iu/l and transaminase from 80 to 67iu/l). He was re-admitted to hospital 50 days later having drank considerably, with elevated levels of plasma triglycerides and cholesterol which again promptly responded to restriction of alcohol (Fig. 8.19).

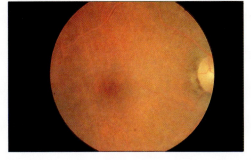

Fig. 8.18 A retinal photograph showing gross lipaemia retinalis, particularly noticeable in the disc vessel at 11 o'clock.

Secondary Hyperlipidaemias

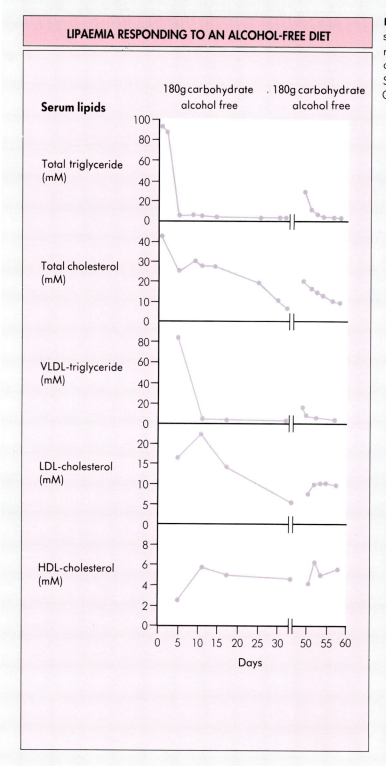

Fig. 8.19 Elevated levels of serum triglycerides, which responded to a restriction of alcohol. Data modified from Stocks J, Holdsworth G, Galton DJ. *Lancet* 1979;**ii**:667.

The adverse response to alcohol intake may have been related to his C-apolipoproteins. Gel electrophoresis showed that he had an excess of apolipoprotein CIII-2 (Fig. 8.20). This observation was clearly shown again on densitometric scans (Fig. 8.21), suggesting that this patient has a mild abnormality of his C-apolipoproteins which are involved in triglyceride transport and which may predispose him to respond to dietary alcohol, by a gross elevation of his plasma lipids.

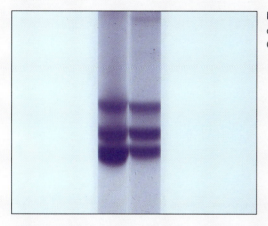

Fig. 8.20 Gel electrophoresis of C-apolipoproteins demonstrating the presence of excess apolipoprotein CIII-2 (lowest band in left-hand track).

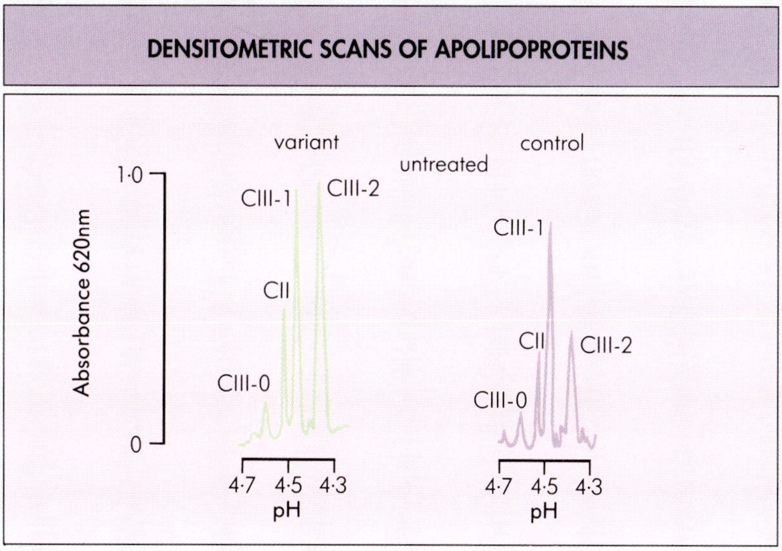

Fig. 8.21 Densitometric scans confirming excess apolipoprotein CIII-2 carried on the triglyceride-rich lipoproteins of the patient.

CHAPTER NINE

Therapy

WHEN TO TREAT HYPERLIPIDAEMIA

Hypercholesterolaemia

The problem with the treatment of hyperlipidaemia due to high levels of cholesterol, is the definition of the 'normal' level of blood cholesterol. There is a wide variation in the mean value of blood cholesterol levels amongst different countries (see *Fig. 4.3*). This variation may be accounted for by both genetic and environmental factors, such as the amount of animal fats that the population consumes. Whether all countries should try to maintain the blood cholesterol at the level of, for example, the rural Japanese, who have a comparably low incidence of coronary artery disease, needs to be established. Classic dietary studies by Ancel Keys and colleagues have shown a striking relationship between the percentage of calories from dietary fats and the levels of blood cholesterol amongst groups as diverse as Japanese farmers and Europeans from South Africa (Fig. 9.1).

To attempt to eliminate the genetic components of hyperlipidaemia, studies of Japanese men consuming traditional diets in Southern Japan and more Europeanized diets in Los Angeles, have been carried out, and again the consumption of animal fats bears a striking relationship with levels of blood cholesterol (Fig. 9.2). Thus, the problem of when to treat hypercholesterolaemia depends upon which group of people is considered, and where they live. One way to simplify this problem is to observe the curvilinear relationship between levels of blood cholesterol and the incidence of coronary heart disease, as in the Multiple Risk Factor Intervention Trial (MRFIT) (Fig. 9.3).

When to Treat Hyperlipidaemia

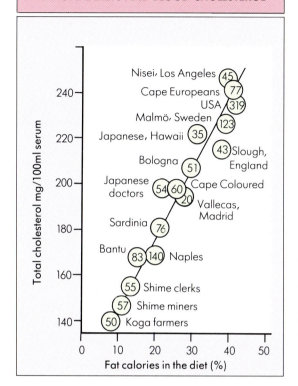

Fig. 9.1 Mean percentage of calories from dietary fats, and levels of total blood cholesterol in 1,288 healthy men, aged 40–49. Data modified from Keys A et al. Ann Int Med 1958;**48**:83.

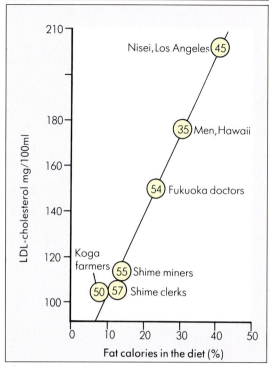

Fig. 9.2 Mean percentage of calories from dietary fats, and levels of LDL-cholesterol in the blood of Japanese men, aged 40–49, in Japan, Hawaii, and Los Angeles. Data modified from Keys A et al. Ann Int Med 1958;**48**:83.

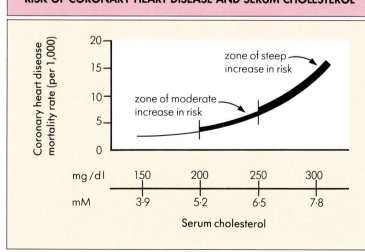

Fig. 9.3 Curvilinear relationship between levels of blood cholesterol and risk of coronary heart disease in 361,000 men screened for entry into the Multiple Risk Factor Intervention Trial (MRFIT). Data modified from Martin MJ, Hulley SB, Browner SL et al. Lancet 1986;**ii**:933.

Individuals with blood cholesterol levels of less than 5.2mM (200mg/dl) are at very low risk of developing coronary heart disease; this risk increases moderately at blood cholesterol levels of 5.2–6.5mM (200–250mg/dl), and increases further at levels of more than 6.5mM (250mg/dl). It seems reasonable therefore to treat individuals who have a high-risk profile (for example, those who have a family history of coronary artery disease or diabetes, or those with previous angina or infarction), if their level of blood cholesterol is above 5.2mM (200mg/dl). Individuals who have a low-risk profile require treatment only if their levels of blood cholesterol are above 6.5mM (250mg/dl). Certain conditions are known to predispose to coronary artery disease and can produce a high-risk profile (Fig. 9.4). Levels of cholesterol which require treatment, as related to age groups (as recommended by a USA 'consensus' conference) are shown in Fig. 9.5. Other National Conferences have assembled and given broadly similar values of levels of blood cholesterol which require treatment.

Hypertriglyceridaemia

The levels of triglycerides which require treatment are easier to establish than those of cholesterol since normal ranges, which are age- and sex-related, can be used (as for blood glucose) throughout world populations.

In middle-aged men in Western societies, levels of triglycerides above 2mM (177mg/dl) can be considered for dietary therapy, depending on HDL levels, and those above 4mM (354mg/dl) for diet and drug therapy.

FACTORS AFFECTING THERAPY OF HYPERLIPIDAEMIA	
Modifiable risk factors	**Other factors**
hypertension	family history of coronary heart disease or peripheral vascular disease
cigarette smoking	
diabetes mellitus	personal history of early onset coronary heart disease
obesity	
alcohol intake	male sex

Fig. 9.4 Factors affecting therapy of hyperlipidaemia.

LEVELS OF CHOLESTEROL REQUIRING TREATMENT ACCORDING TO THE RECOMMENDATIONS OF A USA CONSENSUS CONFERENCE				
Age (years)	Moderate risk		High risk	
	mg/dl	mM	mg/dl	mM
20–29	>200	5.17	>220	5.69
30–39	>220	5.69	>240	6.21
>40	>240	6.21	>260	6.72

Fig. 9.5 Levels of cholesterol which require treatment according to the recommendations of a USA consensus conference. *J Am Med Assoc* 1985;**253**: 2080.

HOW TO TREAT HYPERLIPIDAEMIA

Diets used to treat hyperlipidaemia

In view of the strong dietary influence on levels of blood cholesterol and triglyceride, the general principle of dietary treatment is to reduce the consumption of the relevant nutrient, that is, to reduce dietary cholesterol for hypercholesterolaemia, and neutral fats (triglycerides) for hypertriglyceridaemia. This form of treatment can often work very effectively for hyperlipidaemia with a strong environmental, as opposed to genetic predisposition.

The general principles of the diets used to treat hyperlipidaemia are shown in Fig. 9.6. The patient needs to spend at least half-an-hour with a sympathetic dietitian to discuss his or her current diet, and also the changes which should be made for it to become therapeutic. A diet sheet provided by a doctor in his consulting room, with brief explanations, would in most cases prove ineffective. Follow-up by the dietitian is required in order to encourage and ensure compliance with the diet. Examples of very effective dietary treatments are shown in *Fig. 8.19* (see *Chapter 8*). The other conditions in *Fig. 9.4* must be treated in their own rights to reduce the risk of developing atherosclerosis.

A more detailed account of the diets used for each type of the Fredrickson hyperlipidaemias are shown in Fig. 9.7. It is interesting to find that even the genetically determined hyperlipidaemia of lipoprotein-lipase deficiency (Type I) can be treated effectively by dietary means by withholding long-chain triglycerides in the diet and using short- or medium-chain fats instead. The use of medium-chain fats bypasses the formation of chylomicrons in the intestines (the short-chain fatty acids are absorbed directly into the portal circulation for transport to, and oxidation in the liver) and so chylomicrons will accumulate to a lesser extent in the blood.

THE GENERAL LIPID-LOWERING DIET: NUTRIENT COMPOSITION AND SOURCES

Principle	Sources
decreased total-fat intake and reduction of saturated fats	butter, hard margarine, whole milk, cream, ice cream, hard cheese, cream cheese, visible meat fat, usual cuts of red meat and pork, duck, goose, usual sausage, pastry, usual coffee whiteners, coconut, coconut oil, and palm oil-containing foods
increased use of high protein, low-saturated fat foods	fish, chicken, turkey, veal
increased complex carbohydrate and fruit, vegetable, and cereal fibre, with some emphasis on legumes	all fresh and frozen vegetables, all fresh fruit, all unrefined cereal foods, lentils, dried beans, rice
moderately increased use of polyunsaturated and monounsaturated fats	sunflower oil; corn oil; soya bean oil and products unless hardened (hydrogenated); olive oil
decreased dietary cholesterol	red meats, sweetbreads, kidneys, tongue; eggs (limit to 1–2 yolks per week); liver (limit to twice per month)
moderately decreased sodium intake	salt, sodium glutamate, cheese, tinned vegetables and meats, salt-preserved foods (ham, bacon, kippers), high-salt mineral waters, many convenience foods

Fig. 9.6 The general principles of lipid-lowering diets: Nutrient composition and sources.

Therapy

	Type I	Type II	Type III	Type IV	Type V
Diet prescription	low fat 15–25g/day	low-cholesterol polyunsaturated fat increased	low cholesterol approximately: 20% calories protein 40% calories fat 40% calories carbohydrate	controlled carbohydrate approximately 40% of calories moderately restricted cholesterol	restricted fat 20% of calories controlled carbohydrate 50% of calories moderately restricted cholesterol
Calories	not restricted	not restricted	achieve and maintain 'ideal' weight, that is, reduction diet if necessary	achieve and maintain 'ideal' weight, that is, reduction diet if necessary	achieve and maintain 'ideal' weight, that is, reduction diet if necessary
Protein	total protein intake is not limited	total protein intake is not limited	not limited	not limited other than control of patient's weight	high protein
Fat	restricted to 15–25g/day type of fat important (short-chain triglycerides preferable)	animal-fat intake limited plant-fat intake increased	controlled to 30% calories (polyunsaturated fats recommended in preference to saturated fats)	not limited other than control of patient's weight (polyunsaturated fats recommended in preference to saturated fats)	restricted to 20% of calories polyunsaturated fats to saturated fats
Cholesterol	not restricted	as low as possible	less than 300mg	moderately restricted to 300–500mg	moderately restricted to 300–500mg
Carbohydrate	not limited	not limited	controlled most concentrated sweets are eliminated	controlled most concentrated sweets are eliminated	controlled most concentrated sweets are eliminated
Alcohol	not recommended	may be used with discretion	limited to 2 units/day (substituted for carbohydrate)	limited to 2 units/day (substituted for carbohydrate)	not recommended

Fig. 9.7 Diets used for each type of the Fredrickson hyperlipidaemias.

Medication used to treat hyperlipidaemia: Lipid-lowering therapy

After 2–3 months of dietary therapy, the blood fats may still fail to return to desirable levels, and the use of drugs should be considered. In 1971, only three classes of oral agents were in use, these being the bile acid resins (for example, cholestyramine), the fibrates (for example, clofibrate), and the nicotinates (for example, niacin). There are now six classes of preparations or agents (Fig. 9.8) and their general use for the treatment of hypercholesterolaemia or hypertriglyceridaemia is indicated in Fig. 9.9. The use of hypolipidaemic agents varies widely amongst different countries, with minimal use being found in the UK (Fig. 9.10). The number of prescriptions of

How to Treat Hyperlipidaemia

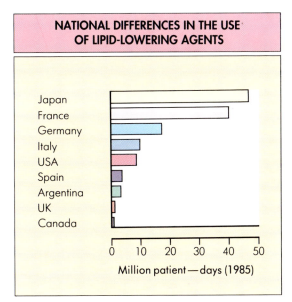

Fig. 9.8 Main classes of agents used in the treatment of hyperlipidaemia.

hypolipidaemic drugs bears no relation to the incidence of hyperlipidaemia in the population, and agents which lower blood fats are least used within the UK when compared to those used to treat other equally common disorders such as diabetes or hypertension (Fig. 9.11).

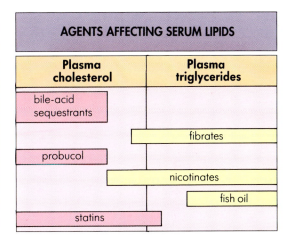

Fig. 9.9 Agents grouped according to whether their predominant action is on serum cholesterol or triglycerides.

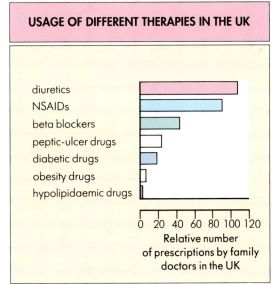

Fig. 9.10 The number of patients treated for one day with lipid-lowering agents in different countries. The number of prescriptions bears no direct relationship with the prevalence of hyperlipidaemia. Modified from Durrington PN. *Hyperlipidaemia: diagnosis and management*. London: Wright, 1989.

Fig. 9.11 The number of prescriptions of lipid-lowering agents in comparison with the use of other drugs in the UK.

Therapy

Bile acid resins

The two most common bile acid resins which are used for treatment of hypercholesterolaemia are cholestyramine and colestipol (Fig. 9.12). These resins bind bile acids in the small intestines and interrupt the enterohepatic circulation of bile acids, so promoting their excretion in the faeces (Fig. 9.13). Bile acids are derived directly from cholesterol, thus allowing its excretion from the body; up to 15g of cholesterol per day may be eliminated in this way. The drugs are not absorbed into the body, therefore systemic side effects do not occur. However, the bile acid resin complex may cause constipation, or occasionally may irritate the colon and produce loose motions or even a mucus diarrhoea; adjustment of the dosage can usually minimize these effects.

The preparations should be taken just before main meals in order to reach the duodenum where the maximum flow of bile acid is likely to occur. They should not be taken under fasting conditions since they will be excreted without binding much to bile acids.

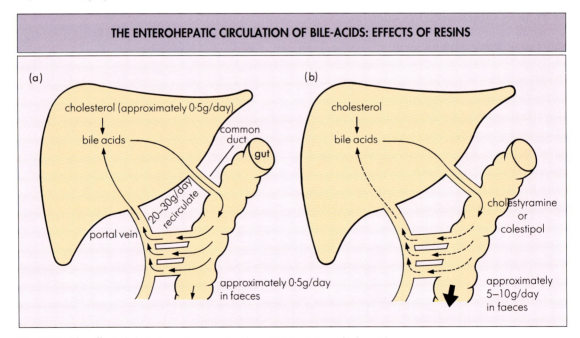

Fig. 9.12 The polymeric structure of bile-acid sequestrants.

Fig. 9.13 The effect of cholestyramine on enterohepatic circulation of bile acids.
(a) Enterohepatic circulation of bile acids. (b) The effect of bile-acid resins on the circulation.

Due to the lack of absorption and systemic side effects, the therapy is suitable for children and teenagers with hypercholesterolaemia, although some prefer not to use them in women who are pregnant. Depending upon the severity of the hypercholesterolaemia and the presence of associated clinical features which may relate to the development of coronary atherosclerosis, up to 2–3 sachets, three times daily, can be taken. During the treatment period, levels of plasma triglyceride may rise slightly due to reasons which are as yet unexplained, but this is not usually a contra-indication.

Plant fibres, such as guar gum, may have a similar action to the resins by binding bile acids more loosely in the intestines, and promoting their excretion in the faeces.

The fibrates

The parent compound of the fibrates is clofibrate, which has some clinically useful derivatives (Fig. 9.14). The mechanism of action of fibrates is still not clearly understood, but it is known that they can induce lipases which clear lipoproteins from the bloodstream (Fig. 9.15). In addition, they may possibly inhibit lipid synthesis in the liver. Fibrates are safe compounds to use, with only rare side effects such as skin rashes and marrow dysplasias. Gemfibrozil was used in the Helsinki Heart Study (see *Chapter 10*), and was shown over a five-year trial period, to lower the levels of LDL-cholesterol and plasma triglyceride, to raise the

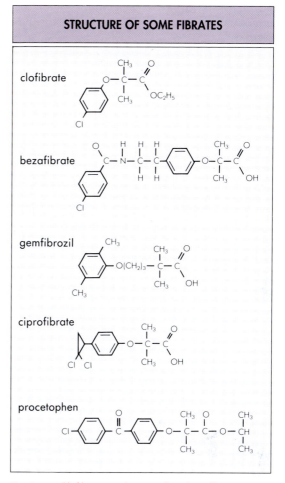

Fig. 9.14 Clofibrate and some of its clinically useful derivatives.

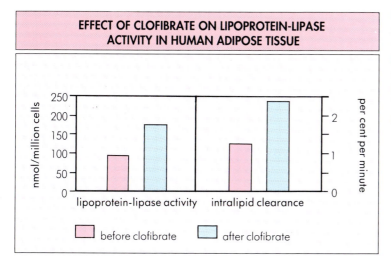

Fig. 9.15 The effect of clofibrate therapy (0.5g, twice daily, for one week) on the activity of lipoprotein lipase in human adipose tissue, and on the clearance of intralipid from the bloodstream. Data modified from Taylor KG, Holdsworth G, Galton DJ. *Lancet* 1977;**ii**:1106.

levels of HDL-cholesterol, and to reduce the incidence of coronary events. Fibrates act synergistically with bile acid resins, and are frequently used in such combinations before attempting to use more potent agents.

The nicotinates

Nicotinic acid (Fig. 9.16a) inhibits the breakdown of intracellular triglycerides to free fatty acids (an antilipolytic action) and hence reduces the recycling of free fatty acids in plasma to the liver (Fig. 9.17). Reduced flux of fatty acids to the liver impairs the synthesis of hepatic triglyceride, and reduces the level of plasma triglycerides. However, the therapeutic dose of nicotinic acid (up to 3–5g per day) is close to the dosage which produces side effects, thereby making the use of the drug difficult. The dose should be built up slowly, starting with as little as 100mg daily. The appearance of vasomotor effects of the skin, such as flushing, sunburn-like rashes, or feelings of prickly heat, indicate that the dosage should be reduced; some of these symptoms can be alleviated using aspirin. Nicotinic acid was used in the Cholesterol-lowering Atherosclerosis Study (CLAS) (see *Chapter 10*) in combination with colestipol, and was shown to be effective in reducing the number of adverse coronary events.

Acipimox is a derivative of nicotinic acid and appears to have fewer side effects, while still retaining a strong antilipolytic action (see *Fig. 9.16b*). Its use in hypertriglyceridaemia and atherosclerosis is under clinical evaluation.

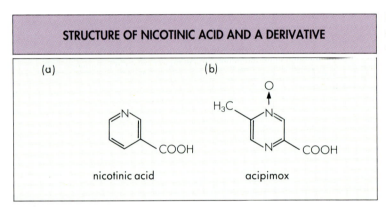

Fig. 9.16 Structure of (a) nicotinic acid (niacin), and (b) one of its derivatives, acipimox.

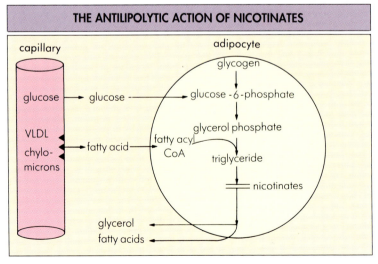

Fig. 9.17 A mechanism of action of nicotinic acid is to inhibit the release of free fatty acids from adipose tissue (antilipolytic action). This reduces the flux of free fatty acids to the liver.

How to Treat Hyperlipidaemia

STRUCTURE OF PROBUCOL

Fig. 9.18 The structure of probucol.

A COMPETITIVE INHIBITOR OF HMGCoA REDUCTASE

(a) compactin (b) HMGCoA

The 'antioxidants'

The 'antioxidant', probucol (Fig. 9.18), lowers the levels of plasma cholesterol by a mechanism which is not yet well established; it may also lower levels of HDL. The drug may have independent anti-atherogenic properties due to its antioxidant properties. It may prevent the oxidative modification of lipoproteins before their incorporation into the fatty streak of the arterial wall.

Probucol appears to be quite safe, and is worthwhile using if more conventional therapies (fibrates and bile acid resins) have failed to lower the levels of blood cholesterol.

The statins

The statins are a very effective group of drugs which directly inhibit cholesterol synthesis in the liver and peripheral tissues. The parent compound, compactin (Fig. 9.19a), is a fungal metabolite which was initially tested for antibacterial activity, but was found to possess cholesterol-lowering properties. Compactin has similarity in structure to the metabolic substrate, HMGCoA, with which it competes for enzyme binding to HMGCoA reductase (Fig. 9.19b). Derivatives of compactin, such as lovastatin, pravastatin, and simvastatin, are shown in Fig. 9.20. These statin derivatives all act

Fig. 9.19 The statins. (a) Compactin. (b) HMGCoA. Note the structural similarity of the side chain of compactin to HMGCoA (an intermediate of cholesterol biosynthesis).

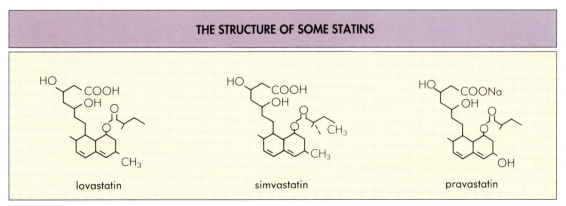

Fig. 9.20 Useful derivatives of compactin.

Therapy

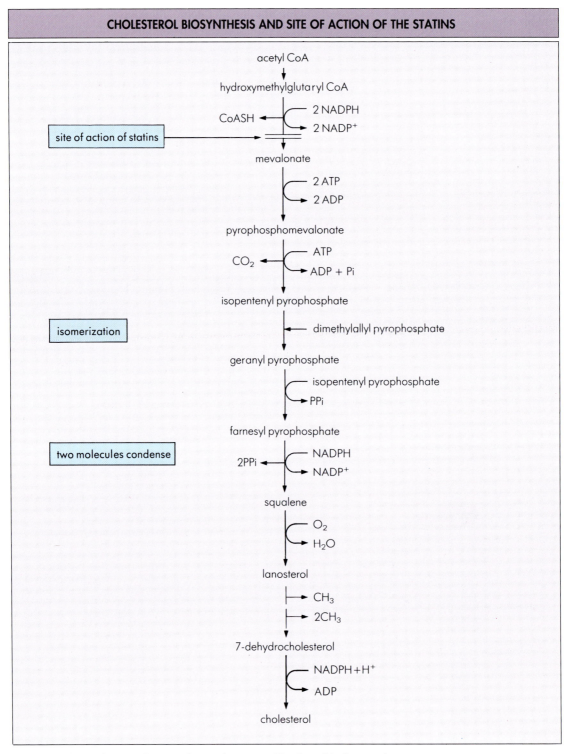

Fig. 9.21 The mechanism of action of statin derivatives. The drugs block a rate-limiting step in the pathway of cholesterol biosynthesis (arrowed).

by competitively inhibiting the rate-determining enzyme, HMGCoA reductase, and by directly inhibiting intracellular pathways of cholesterol synthesis (Fig. 9.21). The rationale for the use of statins is shown in Fig. 9.22 where it is seen that inhibition of cholesterol synthesis (Fig. 9.22b) induces formation of the LDL receptor on the liver-cell membrane, and promotes cholesterol clearance from the bloodstream. Synergistic effects can be obtained with bile acid resins (Fig. 9.22c) which deplete intracellular bile acids and induce more LDL-receptor activity on the cell membrane for removal of LDL-cholesterol from the blood.

Statins are ineffective in homozygous Familial Hypercholesterolaemia, since such patients cannot increase the synthesis and numbers of LDL receptors on their liver-cell membrane. The drugs can be taken after evening meals at doses of up to 40mg per day. Side effects include myopathies and a rise in plasma enzymes from the liver, in which case the dosage should be reduced, or treatment discontinued altogether, depending upon the severity of the complications. The statins should not generally be used in combination with fibrates, since side effects, such as rhabdomyolysis, are more likely to occur.

SYNERGISTIC USE OF STATINS AND BILE-ACID SEQUESTRANTS

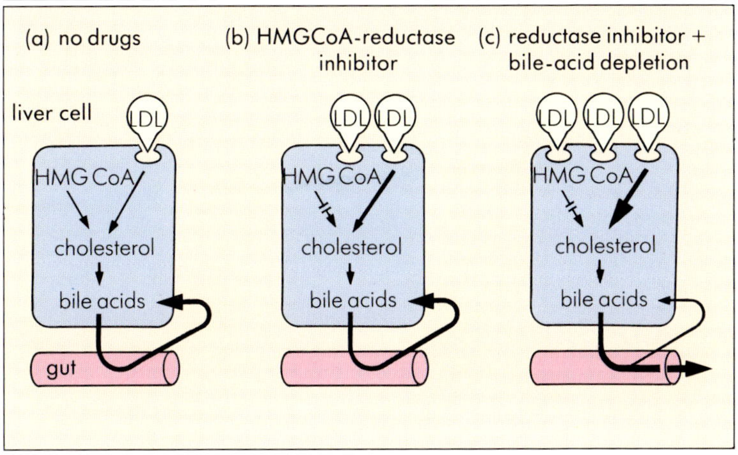

Fig. 9.22 Rationale for the use of an inhibitor of HMGCoA reductase, alone, or in combination with a bile acid resin which induces hepatic LDL-receptor expression and thus lowers plasma levels of LDL. Modified from Brown MS, Goldstein JL. *Sci Am* 1984;**251**:58.

STRUCTURE OF FATTY ACIDS IN MARINE OILS WITH THERAPEUTIC EFFECTS

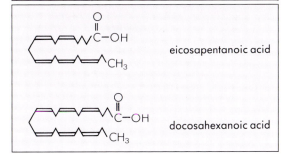

Fig. 9.23 The structure of the long-chain polyunsaturated fatty acids commonly found in some fish oils that therapeutically reduce the plasma concentrations of triglycerides.

Marine oils

Marine oils contain polyunsaturated fatty acids, such as eicosapentanoic acid, which are found at high concentrations in fish (Fig. 9.23). For reasons that are still not clear, marine oils reduce the levels of plasma triglycerides, and can be quite useful in the treatment of moderate to severe hypertriglyceridaemia; levels of plasma cholesterol are also occasionally lowered. The dosage required for treatment is between 4 and 8g per day. Marine oils are naturally occurring fatty acids, and they are generally not toxic. Changes in platelet aggregation or bleeding time might be observed, but this may be beneficial in that intravascular thrombosis may thus be impaired. Marine oils are currently under trial to see if they can prevent coronary artery thrombosis.

Therapy

Summary of the drugs used in hyperlipidaemia

A summary of the properties of some of the more commonly used drugs in the treatment of the hyperlipidaemias is presented in Fig. 9.24. In terms of practice, the general steps used in St Bartholomew's Lipid Clinic to manage a patient with hyperlipidaemia, are shown in Fig. 9.25.

SUMMARY OF THE MAJOR DRUGS USED FOR LOWERING PLASMA LIPIDS					
Drugs	Reduce risk of coronary heart disease	Long-term safety	Maintaining adherence	LDL-cholesterol lowering (%)	Special precautions
Cholestyramine, colestipol	yes	yes	requires considerable education	10–15	can alter absorption of other drugs, for example, antibiotics, diuretics can increase triglyceride levels should not be used in patients with hypertriglyceridaemia
Nicotinic acid	yes	yes	requires considerable education	15–30	test for hyperuricaemia, hyperglycaemia, and liver-function abnormalities
Lovastatin	not proven	not established	relatively easy	25–45	moniter for liver-function abnormalities and myopathies
Gemfibrozil	yes	preliminary evidence satisfactory	relatively easy	5–15	may increase LDL-cholesterol in hypertriglyceridaemic patients should not be used in patients with gallbladder disease
Probucol	not proven	yes	relatively easy	10–15	lowers HDL-cholesterol (significance of this has not been established) prolongs QT interval
Fish oils	not proven	not established	relatively easy	5–10	can prolong bleeding time

Fig. 9.24 Properties of some of the more commonly used drugs for the treatment of hyperlipidaemias.

How to Treat Hyperlipaemia

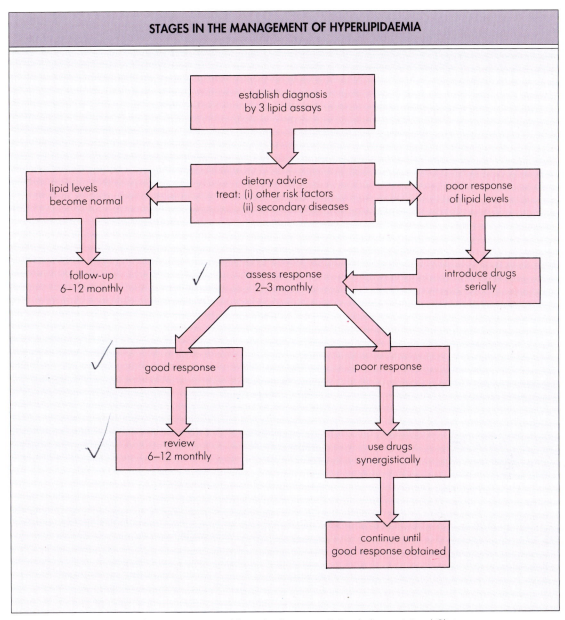

Fig. 9.25 Steps involved in the management of hyperlipidaemia at St Bartholomew's Lipid Clinic.

Drug interactions: Adverse drug effects

Some drugs which are currently used in clinical practice, have been shown to produce a rise in the levels of blood lipids. These drugs include antihypertensive agents, corticosteroids, oral contraceptives, some histamine-receptor blocking agents, and retinoids which are used for dermatological conditions.

Antihypertensive drugs

The thiazide diuretics and beta-adrenergic blocking agents have been incriminated as hyperlipidaemic agents; for example, long-term use of beta-blockers can be associated with a 15–30% increase in serum triglycerides, and a decrease of up to 10% of HDL-cholesterol. The mechanism of this effect is not clear but has been used to explain the

Therapy

EFFECTS OF HYPOTENSIVE DRUGS ON SERUM LIPIDS AND LIPOPROTEINS			
	Cholesterol	Triglyceride	HDL
Diuretics thiazides spironolactone	↑ ±	↑ ±	↔
Beta blockers without SA with SA	↔ ↔	↑ ↔	↓ ↔
Sympatholytics prazosin clonidine methyldopa	↓ ↓ ↔	↔ ↔ ↔	± ↔ ↔
ACE inhibitors	↔	↔	↔
Calcium antagonists	↔	↔	↔
SA = sympathomimetic activity ACE = angiotensin-converting enzyme			

Fig. 9.26 The effects of hypotensive drugs on serum lipids and lipoproteins.

poor effects of antihypertensive treatment in trials for reducing the incidence of coronary heart disease. This has led to the proposal that other agents, such as the angiotensin-converting enzyme (ACE) inhibitors, or calcium-channel antagonists, may be more beneficial than the beta-blockers. The latter should be prescribed with caution to patients who are known to be hyperlipidaemic. The effects of antihypertensive drugs on serum lipids and lipoproteins are summarized in Fig. 9.26.

Corticosteroids

Corticosteroids, a class of drugs which are used in the long-term treatment of asthma and rheumatoid arthritis, and as immunosuppressants after renal or other transplants, can cause a marked rise in plasma triglycerides, and a fall in HDL-cholesterol. These changes may be, in part, responsible for the macrovascular disease which occurs after renal transplantation. The mechanism of the effect of steroids may be mediated by insulin resistance, impaired glucose tolerance, and the subsequent change in free fatty-acid flux (see *Fig. 8.8*) seen in cases of impaired glucose tolerance.

Oral contraceptive agents

Women on long-term administration of the oral contraceptive pill have been shown to have higher serum cholesterol and triglyceride levels than women who do not take such preparations. Occasionally, oral contraception can provoke a massive hypertriglyceridaemia, sufficiently severe to precipitate acute pancreatitis. These effects have been attributed to the oestrogen components of the pill, and women with mild hyperlipidaemia are best advised to use such agents for not longer than 12 months.

Other drugs

Patients who have undergone renal transplant and are using cyclosporin, have been shown to have increased levels of serum cholesterol. This may be due to the hepatotoxic effects of the drug, which impair liver uptake of lipoprotein-cholesterol. Epileptics who are taking phenytoin can have increased levels of HDL, and similar effects have been reported with barbiturates and cimetidine. Other adverse effects of drugs on the levels of blood lipids may occur, and hyperlipidaemic patients should be reviewed carefully; any suspect drug should be discontinued or changed to see if the lipid levels fall.

Surgical measures for hyperlipidaemia: Ileal bypass surgery

Partial ileal bypass surgery can be a useful procedure for severe hypercholesterolaemia which is resistant to drug action, or for patients who cannot tolerate large amounts of hypolipidaemic drugs. The operation involves bypass of the terminal ileum, the site of reabsorption of the bile salts (Fig. 9.27). A surgical interruption of the enterohepatic circulation of bile acids occurs (see *Fig. 9.13*), and up to 15g per day of cholesterol can be excreted in the faeces. The response of plasma cholesterol to such a procedure is dramatic. Six patients with heterozygous Familial Hypercholesterolaemia, who have undergone partial ileal bypass surgery in the St Bartholomew's Lipid Clinic, are presented in Fig. 9.28. Unfortunately, the fall in the levels of plasma cholesterol is not always maintained since the liver starts to augment its synthesis of cholesterol, which tends to restore plasma levels of cholesterol. However, the amount of drug that a heterozygous hypercholesterolaemic patient needs to take can be reduced after ileal bypass. The main side effect of the operation is watery diarrhoea due to irritation by the bile salt load that passes through the colon. In rare cases when this becomes too severe, the bypass can be restored to normal. Malabsorption of fat-soluble vitamins may complicate bypass surgery, and patients may require replacement therapy with vitamin B_{12}.

PARTIAL ILEAL BYPASS SURGERY

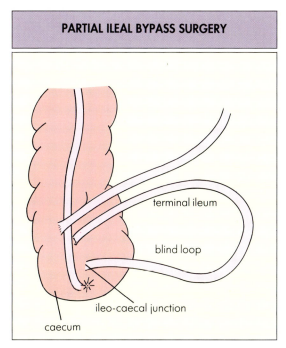

Fig. 9.27 Partial ileal bypass used as a surgical means of interrupting the enterohepatic circulation of the bile salts.

Plasma exchange and LDL-apheresis

Plasma exchange (see *Chapter 2*), or selective binding of LDL-lipoproteins to solid-support materials, as in LDL-apheresis, can be undertaken in specialist hospitals in order to reduce the circulating levels of LDL-lipoproteins in severe hypercholesterolaemia. These procedures are primarily used in homozygous Familial Hypercholesterolaemia.

THE EFFECTS OF PARTIAL ILEAL BYPASS

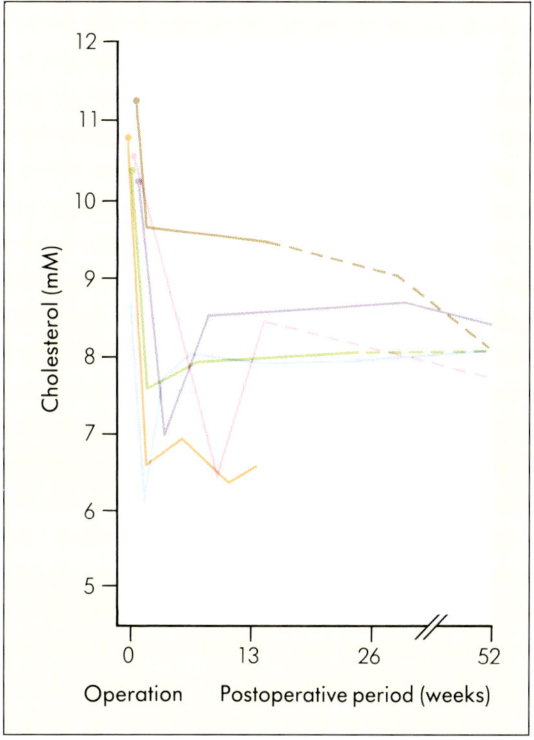

Fig. 9.28 The response of plasma cholesterol to partial ileal bypass in patients with heterozygous Familial Hypercholesterolaemia.

CHAPTER TEN

Intervention Trials

Is the treatment for hyperlipidaemia effective? Fig. 10.1 shows a stepwise relationship between coronary artery disease and levels of serum cholesterol and diastolic blood pressure. If either of the latter is reduced, does the incidence of coronary artery disease fall too? Many clinical trials which

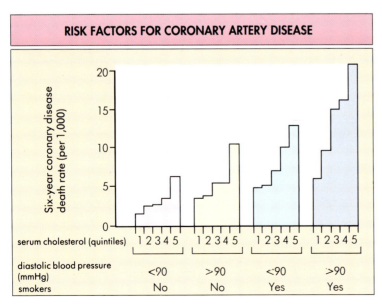

Fig. 10.1 Increased risk of coronary artery disease with increasing levels of cholesterol and blood pressure in men aged 35–57 at entry. Data modified from Stamler J, Wentworth D, Neaton JD. *J Am Med Assoc* 1986;**256**:2823.

have been carried out on subjects with no previous arterial disease (primary prevention trials), or patients with already established arterial disease (secondary prevention trials), have addressed the issue of whether the rate of coronary artery disease will fall if levels of serum cholesterol and diastolic blood pressure are reduced. Almost all the lipid-lowering trials show the same trend, namely, that a fall in levels of blood cholesterol reduces the rate of coronary artery disease. Of these trials, the Lipid Research Clinics Study, the Helsinki Heart Study, and the Cholesterol-lowering Atherosclerosis Study, are some of the most convincing.

THE LIPID RESEARCH CLINICS STUDY

The Lipid Research Clinics Study (a primary prevention trial), using cholestyramine (8g, three times daily) as the active agent, was conducted for seven years on 3,800 middle-aged men from 10 North American lipid clinics. The results show an approximate 12% fall in levels of total cholesterol, very little change in levels of HDL-cholesterol or plasma triglyceride, and approximately 20% reduction in coronary events (defined as fatal or nonfatal infarction, new angina, or development of an abnormal exercise ECG) in the drug-treated group (Fig. 10.2).

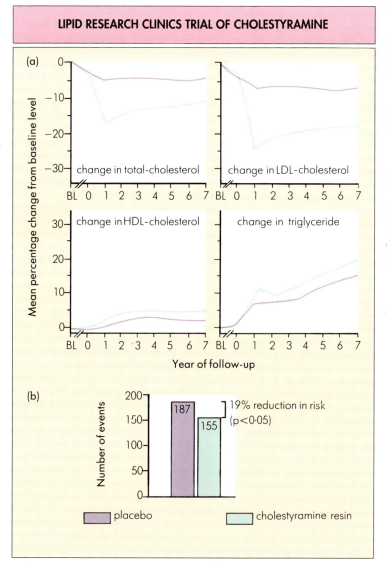

Fig. 10.2 The Lipid Research Clinics Trial: (a) Mean yearly plasma lipid levels for cholestyramine- and placebo-treated men. On the horizontal axis, BL represents the baseline (prediet) period and 0 years represents the three-month interval between the initiation of the Lipid Research Clinics diet and study medication. Year 1 is the average of visits 7 through 13, and each year thereafter represents an average of six visits. (b) Comparison of primary end points occurring in the cholestyramine- and placebo-treated groups. Data modified from Lipid Research Clinics Coronary Prevention Trial. *J Am Med Assoc* 1984;**251**:365.

Intervention Trials

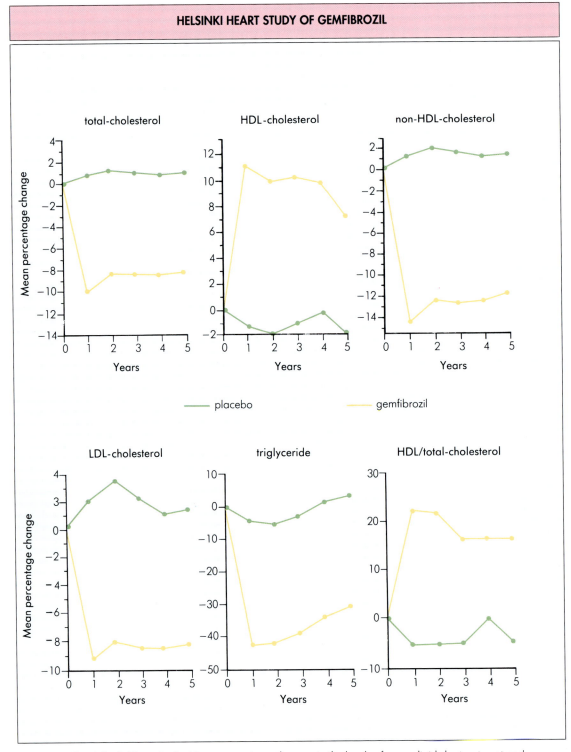

Fig. 10.3 The Helsinki Heart Study: Mean percentage changes in the levels of serum lipids by treatment and time. Data modified from Frick MH, Elo O, Haape K et al. N Engl J Med 1987;**317**:1237.

THE HELSINKI HEART STUDY

The Helsinki Heart Study (a primary prevention trial) was conducted for six years at lipid clinics in Finland, comparing the use of the active agent, gemfibrozil (see *Chapter 9*) in approximately 2,000 men, with the use of placebo in a further 2,000 men. A 10% fall in the levels of (LDL-)cholesterol, an 11% rise in the levels of HDL-cholesterol, and a 40% fall in the levels of plasma triglyceride, were recorded (Fig. 10.3). There was a significant difference in the cumulative incidence of coronary events, defined as fatal or nonfatal infarction, between gemfibrozil- and placebo-treated groups, with an overall 34% reduction in the rate of ischaemic heart disease in the drug-treated group (Fig. 10.4).

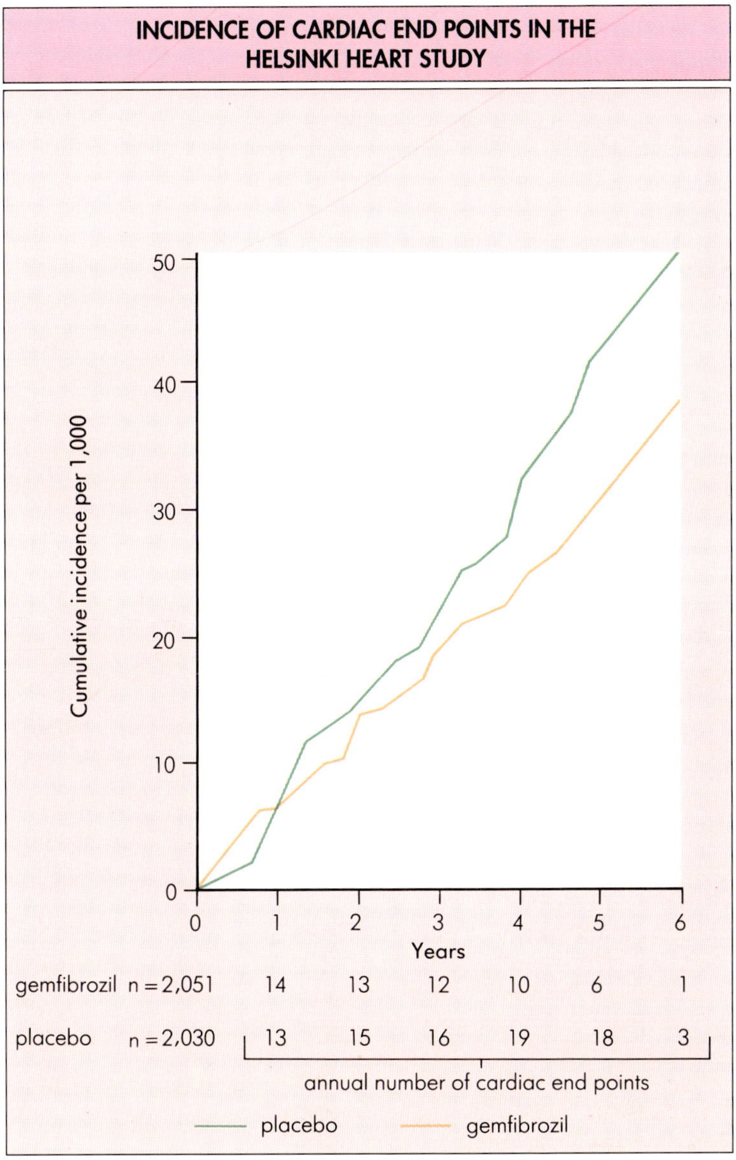

Fig. 10.4 The Helsinki Heart Study: Cumulative incidence (per 10,000) and annual number of cardiac end points, according to treatment group and time. Data modified from Frick MH, Elo O, Haapa K *et al. N Engl J Med* 1987;**317**:1237.

INCIDENCE OF CARDIAC END POINTS IN THE HELSINKI HEART STUDY

	0	1	2	3	4	5	6
gemfibrozil n = 2,051		14	13	12	10	6	1
placebo n = 2,030		13	15	16	19	18	3

annual number of cardiac end points

THE CHOLESTEROL-LOWERING ATHEROSCLEROSIS STUDY

The Cholesterol-lowering Atherosclerosis Study (CLAS) was a placebo-controlled trial using colestipol and nicotinic acid in 162 nonsmoking men aged 40–59, who had undergone coronary by-pass surgery. The end points of the study were the appearances of coronary angiography, assessed objectively after two years of treatment. A 26% reduction in levels of total cholesterol, a 43% reduction in levels of LDL-cholesterol, and a 37% increase in levels of HDL-cholesterol, were observed in the drug-treated group. These results were associated with a significant reduction in the average number of atherosclerotic lesions that progressed per subject ($p<0.03$), and in the percentage of subjects with new atheroma formation in native coronary arteries ($p<0.03$). Deterioration in overall coronary status was significantly less in the subjects in the drug-treated group than those in the placebo group ($p<0.01$) (Fig. 10.5).

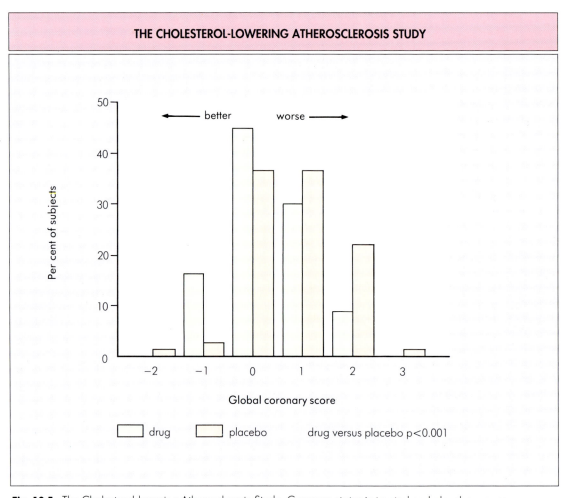

Fig. 10.5 The Cholesterol-lowering Atherosclerosis Study: Coronary status in treated and placebo groups assessed from coronary angiographic appearances (assessed by objective criteria). Deterioration in overall coronary status was significantly less in drug-treated subjects than in placebo-treated subjects. Data modified from Blankenhorn DH, Nessin SA, Johnson RL et al. J Am Med Assoc 1987;**257**:3233.

OTHER TRIALS

A brief summary of some other trials is presented in Fig. 10.6. Although there is a widespread variation in results, most trials show that a reduction in the levels of blood cholesterol, by whatever means, is accompanied by a reduction in coronary events, thereby strongly supporting the rationale of lipid-lowering therapy to prevent coronary artery disease. A strategy to aid prevention of atherosclerosis is described in Fig. 10.7 and might be expected to yield the results of a decline in coronary mortality as shown in *Figs. 4.11* and *4.12* (see *Chapter 4*) for countries such as the USA or Australia; for example, in the femoral angiograms shown in Fig. 10.8, it can be seen that lowering the levels of blood cholesterol for 22 months has improved atherosclerotic lesions of the arterial wall; the thickened and irregular arterial wall becomes thinner and more regular after treatment with cholestyramine, thus implying that local atheromatous deposits may have regressed.

LIPID-LOWERING TRIALS FOR THE PREVENTION OF CORONARY HEART DISEASE

Trial	Treatment	Duration (years)	Change in serum lipids			Outcome
			Total cholesterol (%)	Triglyceride (%)	HDL-cholesterol (%)	
Primary						
Oslo	diet and antismoking	5	−20	−29	—	45% ↓ all CHD
WHO	clofibrate	5.3	−9	—	—	25% ↓ nonfatal CHD 25% ↑ total mortality
LRC–CPPT	cholestyramine	7	−12	+17	+6	19% ↓ all CHD
Helsinki Heart Study	gemfibrozil	5	−9	−35	+9	34% ↓ all CHD
Los Angeles VA	diet	8	−13	—	—	3.2% ↓ all CHD
Finnish Diet Study	diet	6	−12 to −18	—	—	8% ↓ all CHD
Secondary						
Coronary Drug Project	nicotinic acid	6	−9	−27	—	12% ↓ fatal CHD * 11% ↓ total mortality *
Stockholm Trial	clofibrate + nicotinic acid	5	−13	−19	—	36% ↓ fatal CHD 26% ↓ total mortality
Mean change			−12	−19	+7.5	23% ↓ CHD

CHD = coronary heart disease; LRC–CPPT = Lipid Research Clinics – Coronary Primary Prevention Trial;

* = after 15 years

Fig. 10.6 Summary of some prevention trials.

Intervention Trials

PREVENTION OF ATHEROSCLEROSIS

Identify susceptible person

Low-fat diets

Treat : hypertension
　　　　obesity
　　　　lipaemia
　　　　diabetes

Stop smoking

Fig. 10.7 A practical strategy to aid the prevention of atherosclerosis.

In the UK, 20 million working days are lost each year due to ischaemic heart disease; this is more than the number of days lost due to influenza or arthritis, making an impressive case for reducing levels of blood cholesterol to prevent arterial disease.

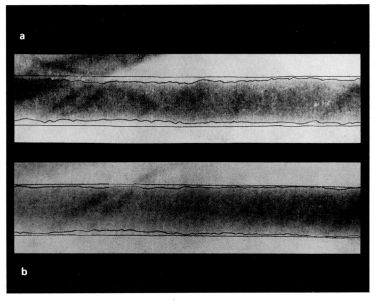

Fig. 10.8 Femoral angiograms showing the effect on atherosclerotic lesions of lowering blood cholesterol levels for 22 months. (a) Before treatment. (b) After treatment with cholestyramine. Note the improvement of the endothelial irregularity after treatment.

CHAPTER ELEVEN
The Lipid Clinic

A lipid clinic sited within a hospital can provide several advantages, these being the availability of specialist advice from a trained physician, and access to laboratory facilities for measurement of plasma lipids and lipoproteins; cardiological referral is also facilitated. Severely affected patients, or those responding poorly to therapy, may require permanent follow-up in the clinic, but many others can be referred back to their GPs for long-term supervision. Annual or bi-annual visits to the lipid clinic for further assessment may be justified in the severer cases.

The lipid clinic deals with a range of problems related to the regulation of blood lipids. Special facilities (Fig. 11.1) at the lipid clinic should include a dietitian to provide initial and follow-up advice to all patients. An Ames analyser machine can provide immediate cholesterol measurements (Fig. 11.2). The availability of these measurements can be useful to guide therapy and, if lipid levels are under satisfactory control, may be encouraging for patients whilst they attend the clinic. A variety of self-help societies now also exist, and educational leaflets and booklets which can give patients a better understanding of the problem, and advice on what to do to achieve better lipid control, are available (Fig. 11.3).

SPECIAL FACILITIES AT THE LIPID CLINIC
dietitian
Reflotron machine
educational booklets
computerization

Fig. 11.1 Special facilities at the lipid clinic for the regulation of blood lipids.

The Lipid Clinic

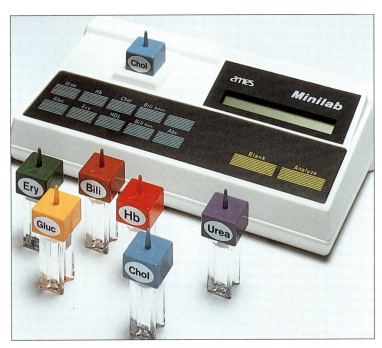

Fig. 11.2 Ames analyser used to provide immediate cholesterol measurements.

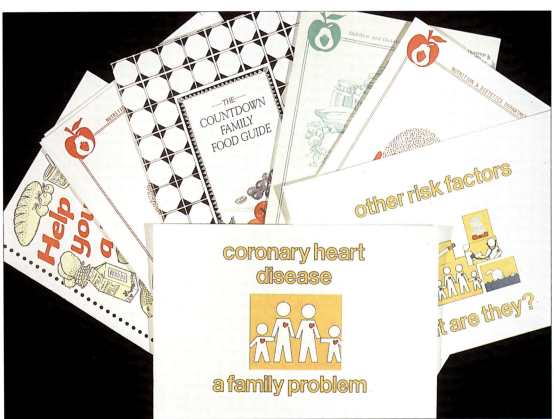

Fig. 11.3 Education leaflets and booklets on lipid control.

Much of the work in the lipid clinic runs on fairly predictable lines, and the clinic is very amenable to computerization. A personal computer is quite sufficient to run a standard-sized clinic. Clinical data can be stored using simple clinical proforma sheets (Fig. 11.4). Letters to GPs can be generated from the stored information to provide regular up-dates on the progress of patients. Furthermore, it is much easier to review the rates of development of atherosclerotic complications and the effects of different therapies on these, when the clinic population is computerized.

Provisions for long-term follow-up can be made in the usual way but will be greatly assisted when simple tests for monitoring blood lipids at home are available. This will allow clinic appointments to be made only at a time when the control of lipid levels has become inadequate. Coping with any chronic disorder is difficult for patients, and the lipid clinic can provide support to continue their efforts to maintain good lipid control.

SCREENING FOR HYPERLIPIDAEMIA

Should the lipid clinic provide a base for screening the entire population for hyperlipidaemia? In view of the frequency of this cardiovascular risk factor, and the reliable means which are now available for its treatment, it would clearly be a desirable option. Ideally, every adult should have serum lipids measured before reaching the age of 25.

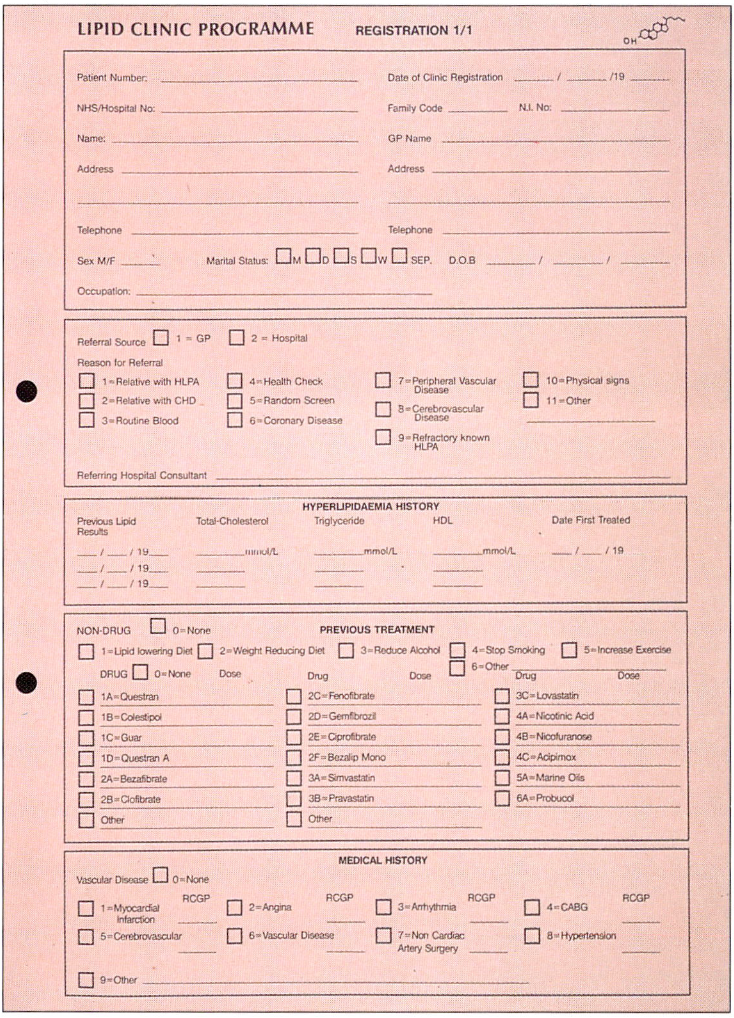
LIPID CLINIC PROGRAMME REGISTRATION 1/1

Patient Number: Date of Clinic Registration / /19
NHS/Hospital No: Family Code N.I. No:
Name: GP Name
Address Address
Telephone Telephone
Sex M/F Marital Status: M D S W SEP. D.O.B / /
Occupation:

Referral Source 1 = GP 2 = Hospital
Reason for Referral
1=Relative with HLPA
2=Relative with CHD
3=Routine Blood
4=Health Check
5=Random Screen
6=Coronary Disease
7=Peripheral Vascular Disease
8=Cerebrovascular Disease
9=Refractory known HLPA
10=Physical signs
11=Other
Referring Hospital Consultant

HYPERLIPIDAEMIA HISTORY
Previous Lipid Results / /19 / /19 / /19
Total-Cholesterol mmol/L
Triglyceride mmol/L
HDL mmol/L
Date First Treated / /19

PREVIOUS TREATMENT
NON-DRUG 0=None
1=Lipid lowering Diet 2=Weight Reducing Diet 3=Reduce Alcohol 4=Stop Smoking 5=Increase Exercise 6=Other
DRUG 0=None Dose Drug Dose Drug Dose
1A=Questran
1B=Colestipol
1C=Guar
1D=Questran A
2A=Bezafibrate
2B=Clofibrate
Other
2C=Fenofibrate
2D=Gemfibrozil
2E=Ciprofibrate
2F=Bezalip Mono
3A=Simvastatin
3B=Pravastatin
Other
3C=Lovastatin
4A=Nicotinic Acid
4B=Nicofuranose
4C=Acipimox
5A=Marine Oils
6A=Probucol

MEDICAL HISTORY
Vascular Disease 0=None
1=Myocardial Infarction RCGP
2=Angina RCGP
3=Arrhythmia RCGP
4=CABG RCGP
5=Cerebrovascular
6=Vascular Disease
7=Non Cardiac Artery Surgery
8=Hypertension
9=Other

Fig. 11.4 Clinical proforma sheets used to store clinical data.

As can be seen in Fig. 11.5, there is wide variation amongst different countries in the screening for hyperlipidaemia. Opponents to this view, point out the major disadvantages of such procedures as the anxiety that such screening can generate in otherwise healthy individuals, and the enormous costs that could be involved in providing therapeutic advice to the large numbers of hyperlipidaemic subjects who would be discovered. Two other approaches have been proposed: the first is lipid screening of patients who visit their GPs for whatever reason, much in the same way that hypertension is detected; and the second approach, as followed at St Bartholomew's Hospital, is to screen individuals who are regarded as being at high risk due to a family history of premature coronary artery disease, or those who have a first-degree relative with proven hyperlipidaemia. The indications for selective screening of this sort are presented in Fig. 11.6. This approach, so far, has not placed an excessive clinical burden on the functioning of lipid clinics.

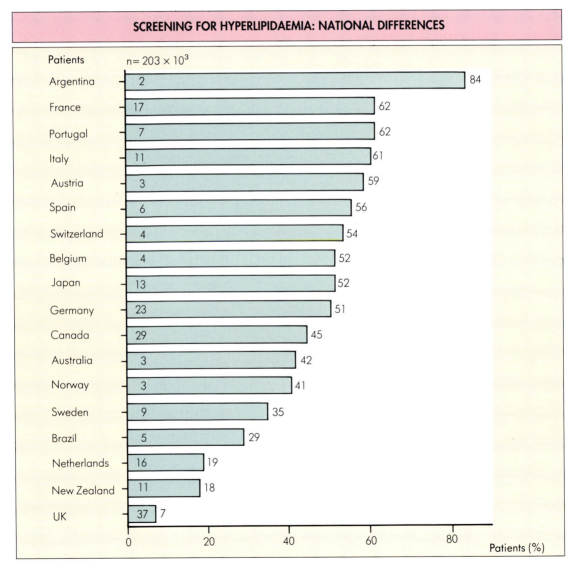

Fig. 11.5 Numbers of healthy subjects screened for hyperlipidaemia in different countries show wide national differences. Data modified from MSD research, personal communication.

SCREENING FOR HYPERLIPIDAEMIA

First-degree relatives of known hyperlipidaemics

Xanthelasma or xanthomata

Corneal arcus before 60 years

Family or personal history of premature arterial disease before 60 years

Hypertension

Diabetes

Chronic renal disease

Fig. 11.6 Indications for screening for hyperlipidaemia.

FUTURE DIRECTIONS

Clinical lipidology can be said to have emerged since 1967 with the introduction of the Fredrickson classification of the hyperlipidaemias. As a result, lipid clinics have been set up on an *ad hoc* basis, generally under the aegis of chemical pathologists, diabetologists, or cardiologists. As a result, there are no clear guidelines for the training of the medical profession to run a lipid service, as, for example, there are for running a diabetic service. Inclusion of lipid metabolism in the undergraduate curriculum, in postgraduate courses, and in refresher courses for cardiologists, diabetologists, and endocrinologists, would clearly help to remedy this. The problems associated with the recruitment of doctors to this specialist field are that no consultant posts (or sessions) are currently designated to run such a lipid service, and that there is no permanent financial support or career structure for junior doctors. Until these matters are rectified, it will be difficult to create more lipid clinics in hospitals which require them, particularly when they have active cardiac and cardiological surgical departments.

Further Reading

Lipid, Lipoprotein Structure, and Metabolism

1. Alberts B, Bray D, Lewis J, Raff M, Roberts K, Watson JD. *Molecular biology of the cell.* New York and London: Garland Inc, 1989.
2. Bierman EL, Oram JF. The interaction of high density lipoproteins with extrahepatic cells. *Am Heart J* 1987;**113**:549–50.
3. Bloomfield VA, Harrington RE. Biophysical chemistry. In: Bloomfield VA, Harrington RE, eds. *Readings from Scientific American.* San Francisco, USA: WH Freeman & Co, 1975:90–9.
4. Brown MS, Goldstein JL. A receptor mediated pathway for cholesterol homeostasis. *Science* 1986;**232**:34–7.
5. Darnell J, Lodish H, Baltimore D. *Molecular cell biology.* San Francisco, USA: WH Freeman & Co, 1988.
6. Hanawalt PC, Hayes RH. The chemical basis of life. In: Hanawalt PC, Haynes RH, eds. *Readings from Scientific American.* San Francisco, USA: WH Freeman & Co, 1978:241–55.
7. Myant NB. *The biology of cholesterol and related steroids.* London: Heinemann Medical, 1981.
8. Piel J. The molecules of life. In: Schwab A, Appenzeller T *et al*, eds. *Readings from Scientific American.* San Francisco, USA: WH Freeman & Co, 1985:50–8.
9. Reichl D, Miller NE. The anatomy and physiology of reverse cholesterol transport. *Clin Sci* 1986;**70**:221–31.
10. Kostner GM. Apolipoproteins and lipoproteins of human plasma. Significance in health and in disease. *Adv Lipid Res* 1983;**20**:1–43.

Inherited Defects of Lipid Metabolism

1. Brunzell JD, Albers JJ, Chait AI, Grundy SM, McDonald GB. Plasma lipoproteins in familial combined hyperlipidaemia and monogenic familial hypertriglyceridaemia. *J Lipid Res* 1983;**24**:147–55.
2. Castelli WP. The triglyceride issue: A view from Framingham. *Am Heart J* 1986;**112**:432–7.
3. Fredrickson DS, Levy RI, Lees RS. Fat transport in lipoproteins — an integrated approach to mechanisms and disorders. *New Engl J Med* 1967;**276**:34–42,94–103, 148–50,215–25,273–81.
4. Galton DJ, Thompson GR. Lipids and cardiovascular disease. In: Galton DJ, Thompson GR, eds. *British Medical Bulletin: Volume 46.* Edinburgh: Churchill Livingstone, 1990:873–959.
5. Rifkind BM, Levy RI. *Hyperlipidaemia: Diagnosis and therapy.* New York: Grune & Stratton, 1977.
6. Stanbury JB, Wyngaarden JB, Fredrickson DS, Goldstein JL, Brown MS. *The metabolic basis of inherited disease.* New York: McGraw–Hill, 1983.

The New Genetics

1. Breslow JL. Genetic regulation of apolipoproteins. *Am Heart J* 1987;**113**:422–7.
2. Bock G, Collins GM. Molecular approaches to human polygenic disease. *CIBA Foundation Symposium 130.* Chichester: J Wiley & Sons, 1987.
3. Galton DJ. *Molecular genetics of common metabolic disease.* London: E Arnold, 1985.
4. Freifelder D. Recombinant DNA. In: Freifelder D, ed. *Readings from Scientific American.* San Francisco, USA: WH Freeman & Co, 1978:4–130.
5. Hartl DL, Clark AG. *Principles of population genetics.* Massachusetts, USA: Sinauer Association, 1989.
6. Utermann G. Apolipoprotein E polymorphisms in health and disease. *Am Heart J* 1987;**113**:433–40.
7. Watson JD, Tooze J, Kurtz DT. Recombinant DNA: A short course. In: Watson JD, Tooze J, Kurtz DT, eds. *Scientific American Books.* New York, USA: WH Freeman & Co, 1983:58–106.
8. Weatherall DJ. *The new genetics and clinical practice.* Oxford, New York, Tokyo; Oxford University Press, 1985.

Epidemiology of Blood Lipids and Atherosclerosis

1. Carlson LA, Bottiger LE. Serum triglycerides, to be or not to be a risk factor for ischaemic heart disease? (the Stockholm Prospective Study). *Atherosclerosis* 1981;**39**:287–91.
2. Castelli WP, Garrison RJ, Wilson RWF, Abbott RD, Kannel WB. Incidence of coronary heart disease and lipoprotein cholesterol levels. The Framingham Study. *J Am Med Ass* 1986;**256**:2835–8.
3. Hjermann I, Byre K, Holme I, Leren P. Effect of diet and smoking intervention on the incidence of coronary heart disease; report from the Oslo Study Group. *Lancet* 1981;**ii**:303–10.
4. Keys A. *Seven countries: A multivariate analysis of death and coronary heart disease.* Cambridge Massachusetts, USA: Harvard University Press, 1980.
5. Lewis B, Chait AI, Wootton IDP *et al.* Frequency of risk factors for ischaemic heart disease in a healthy British population with particular reference to serum lipoprotein levels. *Lancet* 1974;**i**:141–6.
6. Lipid Research Clinics Programme Epidemiology Committee. Plasma lipid distributions in selected North American populations: The Lipid Research Clinics Programme Prevalence Study. *Circulation* 1979;**60**:427–39.
7. Stamler J, Wentworth D, Neaton JD. Is relationship between serum cholesterol and risk of premature death from coronary heart disease continuous or graded? Findings in 356,222 primary screenees of the Multiple Risk Factor Intervention Trial (MRFIT). *J Am Med Ass* 1986;**256**:2823–8.

Complications Related to the Skin and Eye

1. Dodson PM, Galton DJ, Hamilton AM, Blach RK. Retinal vein occlusion and the prevalence of lipoprotein abnormalities. *Brit J Ophthal* 1981;**66**:161–4.
2. Dodson PM, Galton DJ, Winder AF. Retinal vascular abnormalities in the hyperlipidaemias. *Trans Ophthal Soc UK* 1981;**101**:17–21.
3. Durrington PN. *Hyperlipidaemia: Diagnosis and management.* London: Wright, 1989.
4. Mansolf FA. *The eye and systemic disease.* Saint Louis, USA: CV Mosby Co, 1975.
5. Perkins ES, Hansell P. *An atlas of diseases of the eye.* Edinburgh: Churchill Livingstone, 1971.
6. Vaughan D, Asbury T. *General ophthalmology.* Los Altos, California: Lange Medical, 1980.

Further Reading

The Arterial Wall

1. Lusis AJ, Sparkes RS. *Genetic factors in atherosclerosis*. Basle: Karger, 1989.
2. Ross R. The pathogenesis of atherosclerosis. An update. *N Engl J Med* 1986;**314**:488–500.
3. Schlierf G, Morl H. *Expanding in atherosclerosis research*. Berlin: Springer–Verlag, 1987.
4. Steinberg D, Parthasarathy S, Carew TE, Khoo JC, Witztum JL. Beyond cholesterol. Modifications of LDL that increase its atherogenicity. *N Engl J Med* 1989;**320**:915–24.
5. Steinberg D. Lipoproteins and atherosclerosis. A look ahead. *Arteriosclerosis* 1983;**3**:283–301.
6. Suckling KE, Groot PHE. *Hyperlipidaemia and atherosclerosis*. London: Academic Press, 1988.

Secondary Hyperlipidaemias

1. Belfiore F, Galton DJ, Reaven GM. *Diabetes mellitus: etiopathogenesis and metabolic aspects*. Basle: Karger, 1984.
2. Crepaldi G, Tiengo A, Baggio G. *Diabetes, obesity and hyperlipidaemias*. Amsterdam: Excerpta Medica, 1985.
3. Fuller JH, Shipley MJ, Rose G, Jarrett RJ, Keen H. Coronary heart disease risk and impaired glucose tolerance: The Whitehall Study. *Lancet* 1980;**i**:1373–6.
4. James RW, Pometta D. *Dyslipoproteinaemias and diabetes*. Basle: Karger, 1985.
5. Jarrett RJ. *Diabetes and heart disease*. Amsterdam: Elsevier, 1984.
6. Keen H, Jarrett J. *Complications of diabetes*. London: E Arnold, 1982.
7. Marks V, Wright J. *Metabolic effects of alcohol. Clinics in endocrinology and metabolism, volume 7*. London: WB Saunders Co, 1976.
8. Reaven GM, Greenfield MS. Diabetic hypertriglyceridaemia. Evidence for three clinical syndromes. *Diabetes* 1981;**30**:66–75.
9. Reckless JPD, Betteridge DJ, Wu P, Galton DJ. High-density and low-density lipoproteins and prevalence of vascular disease in diabetes mellitus. *Br Med J* 1978;**1**:883–6.
10. Watkins PJ. *Long-term complications of diabetes clinics in endocrinology and metabolism, volume 15*. London: WB Saunders Co, 1986.

Therapy and Trials

1. Blankenhorn DH, Nessim SA, Johnson RL, Sammarco ME, Azen SP, Cashin–Hemphill L. Beneficial effects of combined colestipol–niacin therapy on coronary atherosclerosis and coronary vein bypass grafts. *J Am Med Ass* 1987;**257**:3233–40.
2. Crepaldi G, Gotto AM, Manzato E, Baggio G. *Atherosclerosis VIII*. Amsterdam: Excerpta Medica, 1989.
3. LaRosa JC, Hunninghake D, Bush D, Criqui MH, Getz GS, Gotto AM *et al*. The cholesterol facts: A summary of evidence relating dietary fats, serum cholesterol and coronary heart disease. *Circulation* 1990;**81**:1721–33.
4. Lipid Research Clinics Programme. The Lipid Research Clinics Coronary Primary Prevention Trial Results. The relationship of reduction in incidence of coronary heart disease to cholesterol lowering. *J Am Med Ass* 1984;**251**:365–74.
5. Manninen V, Elo O, Frick H, Haapa K, Heinsalmi P *et al*. Lipid alterations and decline in the incidence of coronary heart disease in the Helsinki Heart Study. *J Am Med Ass* 1988;**260**:641–51.
6. Oliver MF, Healy JA, Morris JN *et al*. A co-operative trial in the primary prevention of ischaemic heart disease using clofibrate. *Br Heart J* 1978;**40**:1069–78.
7. Shepherd J, Packard CJ, Bicker S, Lawrie TDV, Morgan HG. Cholestyramine promotes receptor mediated low density lipoprotein catabolism. *N Eng J Med* 1980;**302**:1219–22.
8. Assman G, Lewis B, Mancini M, Stein *et al*. Strategies for the prevention of coronary heart disease. A policy statement for the European Atherosclerosis Society. *Eur Heart J* 1987;**8**:77–88.
9. Thompson GR, Barbir M, Michishita I, Larkin S. Comparison of plasma exchange and LDL apheresis in the treatment of hypercholesterolaemia. In: Crepaldi G, Gotto AM, Manzato E, Baggio G, eds. *Atherosclerosis VIII*. Amsterdam: Excerpta Medica, 1989:815–8.
10. Miettinen M, Turpeinen O, Karronen MJ *et al*. Effect of cholesterol-lowering diet on mortality from coronary heart disease and other causes. *Lancet* 1972;**ii**:835–8.

Index

Achilles tendon 71
acipimox 109, 112
adipocytes 4–5
alcoholism 25, 93, 100–3
Ames analyser machine 23, 127–8
Analyst measuring instrument 23
angiography, detection of atheroma 88–9
angiotensin-converting enzyme (ACE) inhibitors 118
antihypertensive drugs 117–18
'antioxidants' 109, 113, 116
apolipoprotein-B gene 52
apolipoprotein CII 17
    abnormalities 31
    deficiency 28–30
apolipoproteins 6–7, 12
    disorders see under hyperlipidaemias
    genes 49–51
    genetic diversity 50–2
    rare disorders 42
arcus 32, 39
arterial plaque, development of 88
arterial wall see under atherosclerosis
assays of cholesterol and triglycerides 21–3
atheroma
    detection of 88–92
    development of 87–8
atherosclerosis 84–91
    abnormal storage of triglyceride 44–5
    candidate genes 48
    causes of 24–5, 84–5
    critical areas 86
    detection of 88–92
    development of 87–8
    inheritance of 47–8
    pathogenic factors 47
    prevention of 126

balanced polymorphisms 52–3
barbiturates 118
base-pair mismatch technique 59
beta-adrenergic blocking agents 93, 117–18
bezafibrate 109, 111
bile acid resins 109, 110–11, 116
brain, atherosclerosis 86
'Broad-beta' disease 35–6

calcium-channel antagonists 118
candidate genes 47–8
centrifugation of lipoproteins 9–10
chain packing of lipid molecules 3
cholestasis 93
cholesterol
    agents affecting 109
    coronary heart disease 62, 105–6, 120
    dietary fats 105
    esterification of 18
    levels requiring treatment 106
    lipoproteins 6–7
    measurement of 21–3
    molecular structure 1–2
    national diets 105
    statins 113–15
    transport disorders see under hyperlipidaemias
Cholesterol-lowering Atherosclerosis Study (CLAS) 112, 124
cholesteryl-ester transfer protein (CETP) 19
cholestyramine 109, 110, 116
    research trials 121, 125
Chylomicronaemia syndrome 33–4
chylomicrons 6–8
    composition of 7, 10–12
    separation of 9–11
    sources of 13
cimetidine 118
ciprofibrate 111
circulation of lipoproteins 15–16
clofibrate 109, 111
    research trials 125
clonidine 118
colestipol 109, 110, 116
    research trials 124
Combined Hyperlipidaemia, Fredrickson Type IIb 37–8
compactin 113
computerization of data 129
contraceptive, oral 118
Coronary Drug Project 125
coronary heart disease see under heart disease
corticosteroids 118
cyclosporin 118

diabetes mellitus 25, 93, 94–9
    complications 94
    development of lipid abnormalities 96
    hypertriglyceridaemia 95–6, 98
    retinal-vein occlusion 78
    vascular disease 95
diagnosis of hyperlipidaemia 26
    Type I 27
    Type IIa 38–9
    Type IIb 37
    Type III 35–6
    Type IV 32
    Type V 34
diet, and blood cholesterol 104–5
diets, lipid-lowering 107–8
    research trials 125
differential subtraction angiography (DSA), detection of atheroma 89
directional selection 52–3
diversity, genetic 50–2
DNA polymorphisms 54–7
docosahexanoic acid 115
Doppler ultrasound, detection of atheroma 89–90, 91

Index

drug interactions, causing rise in blood lipid levels 117–18
drug therapy 108–16
   'antioxidants' 109, 113, 116
   bile acid resins 109, 110–11
   fibrates 109, 111–12
   marine oils 109, 115, 116
   nicotinates 109, 112, 116
   statins 109, 113–15, 116
dysgammaglobulinaemia 25

education, leaflets and books 127–8
eicosapentanoic acid 109, 115
electrophoresis of lipoproteins 10
endonucleases 46
enzymes
   abnormal 24, 27–8
   assays of cholesterol and triglycerides 21–3
   in lipid transport 17–19
epidemiology of hyperlipidaemias 60–8
evolution, and genetic variation 52–3
eyelids 69–70
eyes 74–83
   lipaemia retinalis 27, 74
   lipid deposits in cornea 19
   retinal-vein occlusion 78–81
   retinal xanthoma 74–5
   venous thrombosis 75–7

Fabry disease 42
Familial Dyslipoproteinaemia ('Broad-beta' disease), Fredrickson Type III 35–6
Familial (Primary) Hypertriglyceridaemia, Fredrickson Type I 27–31
Familial (Polygenic) Hypertriglyceridaemia, Fredrickson Type IV 32–3
'fat gene' map 48
fatty acids, free 5–6, 15
fatty plaque, origin of 87
feet, lipid deposits 72
fenofibrate 109
fibrates 109, 111–12, 116
'fibre' 109
Finnish Diet Study 125
fish oils 109, 115, 116
'founder' effect 52
Framingham Study, serum lipids and heart disease 63–4
Fredrickson classification of hyperlipidaemias 25–6
   Type I 27–31
   Type IIa 38–9
   Type IIb 37–8
   Type III 35–6
   Type IV 32–3
   Type V 33–4
   see also therapy
fuel
   storage of 3–5

supply, model 5
transport of 5–20
Garrod, Sir Archibald 24
Gaucher's disease 42–3
gemfibrozil 109, 111, 116
   research trials 122–3, 125
gene clusters 49–50
genes, structure of 49–50
genetic drift 52–3
genetic markers 53–7
genetics, new developments 46–59
   candidate genes 47–8
   diversity 50–2
   evolution and genetic variation 52–3
   gene clusters 49–50
   genetic markers 53–7
   methods for studying genetic variation 57–9
glaucoma, neovascular 81
glucose 5
glycerol 4–5
glycogen
   fuel storage 4
   molecular structure 3–4

hands, lipid deposits 44, 71, 73
heart disease
   cholesterol 105–6
   cholesterol levels and blood pressure 120
   lipid levels 61, 63–6
   loss of working days, UK 126
   UK mortality rate 60
   weight 100
   world mortality rates 61
Helsinki Heart Study 111, 122–3
hepatic lipase 13, 18
high-density lipoproteins (HDL) 6–8
   composition of 7, 10–12
   separation of 9–11
   sources of 15
HMGCoA 113–15
hypercholesterolaemia, Fredrickson Type IIa 26, 38–9
   drug therapy 109
   when to treat 104–6
   see also hyperlipidaemias
hyperlipidaemias 24–40
   classification of 25–6
   Combined Hyperlipidaemia, Fredrickson Type IIb 37–8
   Familial Dyslipoproteinaemia ('Broad-beta' disease), Fredrickson Type III 35–6
   Familial (Polygenic) Hypertriglyceridaemia, Fredrickson Type IV 32–3
   Familial (Primary) Hypertriglyceridaemia, Fredrickson Type I 27–31
   Hypercholesterolaemia, Fredrickson Type IIa 38–9
   pool model of 26
   screening for 129–31

Index

secondary (q.v.) 93–103
severe hypertriglyceridaemia (Chylomicronaemia syndrome), Fredrickson Type V 33–4
therapy 104–19
hypertension 78
hypertriglyceridaemia 26
   alcoholism 101
   diabetes mellitus 95–6, 98
   drug therapy 109
   when to treat 106
   see also hyperlipidaemias
hypotensive drugs 117–18
hypothyroidism 25, 93, 94

ileal bypass surgery 118–19
insulin 94
intermediate-density lipoproteins (IDL) 6–8
   composition of 10–12
   separation of 9–11
   sources of 13
intervention trials 120–6
   Cholesterol-Lowering Atherosclerosis Study (CLAS) 124
   Helsinki Heart Study 122–3
   Lipid Research Clinics Study 121
   other 125

Japan
   diet and blood cholesterol 104–5
   mortality rates 61, 67–8
   serum cholesterol 62

kidneys
   atherosclerosis 86
   failure 93
kringles 8

lecithin:cholesterol acyltransferase (LCAT) 15, 18
lipaemia retinalis 27, 33, 74
lipases 13, 16–18
   assays of cholesterol and triglycerides 21–3
lipid clinics 127–31
Lipid Research Clinics Study 121
lipoprotein (a) 8–9
lipoprotein lipase 13, 16–17
   clofibrate 111
   defects of 27–9
lipoproteins 6–16
   cascade 13, 41–2
   circulation of 15–16
   composition of 10–12
   enzymes 17–18
   identification of 9–10
   receptors 19–20
   sources of 13–15
   structure of 6–9
lipolytic cascade of lipoproteins 13
   defects of 41–2
liver, secretion of VLDLs 13, 15–16

Los Angeles VA, research trial 125
lovastatin 109, 116
low-density lipoprotein (LDL) 6–8
   apheresis 119
   composition of 7, 10–12
   receptor 19–20, 115
   receptor mutations 38
   separation of 9–11
   sources of 13
lysolecithin 18
lysosomal storage disorders 42–3

magnetic resonance imaging, detection of atheroma 90–2
malondialdehyde 76–7
marine oils 109, 115, 116
markers, genetic 53–7
men, mortality rates and serum lipids 60–2, 67
methyldopa 118
molecules, lipids 1–3
Moorfields Eye Hospital study 77
mortality rates
   changes in 67–8
   coronary heart disease 61
   sex differences 67–8
   UK 60
Multiple Risk Factor Intervention Trial (MRFIT), coronary heart disease 66
mutations
   and evolution 52–3
   techniques for identifying 57–9
myocardial infarction 38, 39–40, 85

national mortality and morbidity rates see under world
nephrotic syndrome 25, 93
nicofuranose 109
nicotinates/nicotinic acid 109, 112, 116
   research trials 124, 125
Niemann–Pick disease 42
nonlysosomal storage disorders 42, 44–5

obesity 25, 93, 100
oestrogen 25, 117, 118
Oslo Heart Study, risk factors in coronary heart disease 64–5
Oslo, prevention trial 125

pancreatitis 25, 75
pedigree genetics 53, 55–6
peptides, in lipoproteins 6–7, 10–12
phenytoin 118
phosphatidylcholine, molecular structure 2
phospholipids
   in lipoproteins 6–7
   molecular structure 2
photocoagulation treatment, retinal-vein occlusion 79, 81
plasma, and diagnosis (q.v.) of hyperlipidaemia 26
plasma exchange 34–5, 119
plasminogen 8
platelet function in hyperlipidaemia 76–7, 80

Polygenic Familial Hypertriglyceridaemia, Fredrickson Type IV 32–3
polymerase chain-reaction technique 57, 59
polymorphisms, DNA 54–7
pool model for hyperlipidaemias 26
population genetics 53–4, 57
population studies, blood lipids and heart disease 63–6
pravastatin 109, 113
prazosin 118
pregnancy 25
probucol 109, 113, 116
procetophen 111

receptors, lipoproteins 19–20, 115
    LDL-apheresis 119
    mutations 38
Reflotron measuring instrument 22–3
remnant receptor 20
renal failure 93
resins, bile acid 109, 110–11
restriction endonucleases 46
restriction fragment-length polymorphisms (RFLPs) 46–7, 55–7
retina
    lipaemia retinalis 27, 33, 74
    vein occlusion 78–81
    xanthoma 74–5

screening for hyperlipidaemias 129–31
    indications for 131
secondary hyperlipidaemias 93–103
    alcoholism 100–3
    causes of 93
    diabetes mellitus 94–9
    hypothyroidism 94
    obesity 100
severe hypertriglyceridaemia (Chylomicronaemia syndrome), Fredrickson Type V 33–4
sickle-cell anaemia 53
simvastatin 109, 113
skin, lipid deposits 27, 32, 36, 70–3
smoking, cigarettes 106
solubility, lipids 2
Southern blotting technique 56, 57, 58
specialists in lipidology 131
spironolactone 118
statins 109, 113–15, 116
steroid therapy 25, 93, 117
Stockholm Prospective Study, plasma lipids and ischaemic vascular deaths 64
Stockholm Trial 125
storage of fuels 3–5
    disorders of 42–5
strokes 61
surgery 118–19
sympatholytics 118

Tay–Sachs disease (sphingolipidosis) 42
tendons, lipid accumulations 71–2

therapy 104–19
    diets 107–8
    drug interactions 117–18
    factors affecting 106
    medication 108–16
    plasma exchange and LDL-apheresis 119
    stages of 117
    surgery 118–19
    Type I 27–8
    Type IIa 39
    Type IIb 38
    Type III 35
    Type IV 32
    Type V 33
    when to treat 104–6
thiazide diuretics 93, 117–18
β-thromboglobulin 76, 80, 81
training in lipidology 131
transport of fuel 5–20
    defects in see under hyperlipidaemias
    enzymes 17–19
    lipoproteins 6–16
    receptors in lipoprotein catabolism 19–20
triglycerides
    agents affecting 109
    breakdown of 17
    chain packing 3
    fuel storage 3–4
    in lipoproteins 6–7
    measurement of 21–3
    molecular structure 1
    storage disorders 44–5
    transport disorders see under hyperlipidaemias

ultrasound, detection of atheroma 89–90, 91
United Kingdom (UK)
    loss of working days due to ischaemic heart disease 126
    mortality rates 60
    usage of lipid-lowering drugs 109
United States of America (USA)
    diet and blood cholesterol 105
    mortality rates, ischaemic heart disease 67

variation, genetic 50–2
    and evolution 52–3
    methods for studying 57–9
Variegate Porphyria 52
venous thrombosis 75–7
    retina 78–81
very low-density lipoproteins (VLDL) 6–8
    composition of 10–12
    separation of 9–11
    sources of 13–14

weight, and coronary morbidity and mortality 100
    see also obesity
women, mortality rates 68
world
    coronary heart disease 62

Index

    diets and cholesterol levels 105
    mortality rates, heart disease 61, 67–8
    screening for hyperlipidaemia 130
    serum cholesterol 62
    usage of lipid-lowering drugs 109
World Health Organisation (WHO), research trial 125

xanthelasma 69–70
xanthomata 27, 32, 36, 70–2
    intracranial 82–3
    retinal 74–5